'I highly recommend this book to clinicians working with children and families affected by developmental trauma. Its practical application of the MBT-C model and its theoretical depth and commitment to inclusivity make it an invaluable resource for practitioners seeking to enhance their clinical practice. Whether you are a seasoned clinician or new to the field, this book offers a wealth of insights and tools to support your work with traumatized children and their families. By engaging with the book's multidimensional approach—spanning assessment, treatment, and systemic interventions—readers will gain a deeper understanding of the complexities of developmental trauma and the transformative potential of mentalization-based treatment. Above all, this book serves as a testament to the power of compassion and understanding in fostering healing and connection in the lives of children and their families.'

Francine Conway, Ph.D., *Chancellor, Distinguished Professor,*
Rutgers University-New Brunswick

'This outstanding book brings the mentalization-based clinical approach to children and young people fully up to date, significantly broadening its scope and showcasing a vibrant array of interventions. Rich in techniques and practical insights, it offers invaluable guidance for all practitioners working from a developmental perspective—whether with children, adolescents, or adults.'

Professor Peter Fonagy CBE FMedSci FBA FAcSS, *Head of the Division*
of Psychology and Language Sciences

Mentalization-Based Treatment for Developmental Trauma

Mentalization-Based Treatment for Developmental Trauma offers mental health practitioners a transdiagnostic model to support the needs of traumatized children with both internalizing (emotional) and externalizing (behavioural) difficulties, and shows how MBT can be applied to meet the needs of children who have experienced various types of developmental trauma.

This volume includes contributions from global experts in MBT who share their experience of using the method with traumatized children in a range of settings, from individual therapy to group work and work with parents, carers, and the networks around the child. They highlight the benefits of using MBT with different groups, such as children in foster or residential care or those who are refugees. The chapters offer a framework for clinicians to support children to better process and regulate their emotions, highlighting the importance of early intervention as a means of mitigating certain psychopathologies that commonly result from developmental trauma. With clinical vignettes throughout, this book covers different stages of treatment, such as assessment, direct therapy with the child, work with the network, and support for carers and parents.

This book is a vital resource for child counsellors, psychologists, psychoanalysts, and therapists who work with children who have experienced developmental trauma, as well as junior psychologists and child psychiatrists, mental health nurses, social workers, and others working in child mental health services.

Nicole Muller is a child and adolescent psychotherapist and family therapist at Centrum Hecht Opleidingen in Holland, a specialist centre for training of professionals and treatment centre of children, youth and their families, specialized in attachment and trauma disorders. She is a MBT-CYP practitioner, supervisor and trainer.

Emma Morris is a consultant clinical psychologist and MBT-CYP practitioner, supervisor, and trainer based in the UK. She is the founder and co-director of the Multi-Family Project and co-director of the Trauma Recovery

Space, a specialist trauma clinic. She is co-author of *High Conflict Parenting Post Separation: The Making and Breaking of Family Ties* (2020) and *Systemic Multi-Family Therapy: Concepts and Interventions* (2024).

Nick Midgley is a child and adolescent psychotherapist and professor of psychological therapies with children and young people at UCL and Anna Freud, London, UK. His books include *Therapeutic Work for Children with Complex Trauma: A Three-Track Psychodynamic Approach* (2023), *Short-term Psychoanalytic Psychotherapy for Adolescents with Depression: A Treatment Manual* (2016), and *Minding the Child: Mentalization-Based Interventions with Children, Young People and their Families* (2012).

Mentalization-Based Treatment for Developmental Trauma

A Casebook for Working with Children and Their Families

Edited by
Nicole Muller, Emma Morris and Nick Midgley

Routledge
Taylor & Francis Group

LONDON AND NEW YORK

Designed cover image: © Tim Juffermans Studio 071

First published 2025
by Routledge
4 Park Square, Milton Park, Abingdon, Oxon OX14 4RN

and by Routledge
605 Third Avenue, New York, NY 10158

Routledge is an imprint of the Taylor & Francis Group, an informa business

British Library Cataloguing-in-Publication Data
A catalogue record for this book is available from the British Library

ISBN: 978-1-032-71342-7 (hbk)
ISBN: 978-1-032-64603-9 (pbk)
ISBN: 978-1-032-71344-1 (ebk)

DOI: 10.4324/9781032713441

Typeset in Times New Roman
by Taylor & Francis Books

Contents

Illustrations

Figures

Tables

Box

Contributors

Jordan Bate is a clinical psychologist and associate professor at Ferkauf Graduate School of Psychology, Yeshiva University in New York, where she is head of the Attachment and Psychotherapy Process research lab and leads the practicum in psychodynamic child therapy. She is on the voluntary faculty of Lenox Hill Hospital, Northwell Health, where she is co-investigator on a pilot study of the implementation of MBT-CYP in the outpatient clinic. Her research also includes the study of attachment-based and mentalization-focused interventions for families involved in the child welfare system, personality development in adolescence, and training for therapists. She is co-author of *Deliberate Practice for Child and Adolescent Psychotherapy*, and *Working with Parents: A Mentalization Based Approach*. She also maintains a private practice in New York City.

Hazal Çelik is a psychoanalytically oriented therapist with expertise in clinical psychology and developmental psychology. She offers therapy for children, adolescents and adults in her own practice in Istanbul, Turkey.

Natasha Dobrova-Krol is a psychotherapist and researcher in the Child and Family Department at ARQ National Psychotrauma Center, Centrum '45, in the Netherlands. She has experience in trauma-focused psychotherapy and international consultancy, with a demonstrated history in mental health care and international project development, including collaborations with organizations like UNICEF and Eurlyaid. She also runs a private psychotherapy practice. She holds a PhD in child and family studies from Leiden University and a background in clinical psychology and psychodiagnostics from Kyiv State Shevchenko University, Ukraine.

Vincent Domon-Archambault is a clinical psychologist working for the Youth Protection Services at CIUSSS du-Centre-Sud-de-l'Ile-de-Montréal, Quebec, Canada. He co-authored articles concerning a mentalizing approach for children and adolescents who experienced trauma and those who care for them. As a clinician, he works with children and adolescents in rehabilitation centres and foster care.

Karin Ensink is a clinical psychologist and professor of psychology in Canada. She is the director of Mentalization Based Treatment Canada, the founder of a clinic for the treatment of complex trauma, and is an Anna Freud Centre recognized MBT supervisor (child, adolescent, and adult) and trainer (child and adolescent). The author of a number of books on the treatment of children and adolescents, including mentalization-based treatment for children, Karin has published widely on the development of mentalizing, the role of mentalizing as a resilience factor in the context of trauma, and personality disorders in adults, parents, adolescents and children. She has active research collaborations in the UK, US, Italy, Spain, France, Norway and Chile.

Dilara Güvenç is a clinical psychologist from Turkey. Her research focuses on understanding change mechanisms in child psychotherapy. She works at a private clinic in Istanbul, providing therapy to children, adolescents, and adults using a psychodynamic approach.

Sibel Halfon is an associate professor of clinical psychology at Istanbul Bilgi University, Turkey, where she also serves as the director of the clinical psychology master's program. She has several publications on the therapeutic benefits of mentalization-based approaches in child psychotherapy.

Masja Juffermans is a child and adolescent health psychologist at Centrum Hecht in Holland, a specialist centre for the treatment of children, youth and their families with attachment and trauma problems. She is a MBTC practitioner, supervisor and trainer. She is also CEO of her own training centre specialized in MBT-CYP: Centrum Hecht Opleidingen. She combines MBT treatment often with EMDR. She has written several articles about her work with traumatized children and parents.

Norka Malberg is a child and adolescent psychotherapist and adult psychoanalyst, and assistant clinical professor at the Yale Child Study Center, Yale School of Medicine. She is co-author of the books: *MBT-C Time Limited Approach* and *Working with Parents in Therapy: A Mentalization Based Approach*, both published by APA books. She is principal investigator in several pilot studies regarding the application of MBT-C in public mental health services and to working with school age autistic children. She is the director of IMAGINA: Centro de Aplicaciones de la Mentalización, a clinical and teaching center based in Barcelona, Spain.

Nick Midgley is a child and adolescent psychotherapist and professor of psychological therapies with children and young people at UCL and Anna Freud, London, UK. In 2012 he co-edited *Minding the Child: Mentalization-Based Interventions with Children, Young People and their Families* (Routledge), and he was a co-author of *Mentalization-Based Treatment for Children: A Time-Limited Approach* (APA, 2017). He is currently leading a randomized controlled trial of MBT for children with emotional and behavioural difficulties, the ERiC study.

Emma Morris is a consultant clinical psychologist, head of psychological therapy innovation and senior family trauma clinician at Anna Freud, London, UK. In 2020 she co-authored *High Conflict Parenting Post Separation: The Making and Breaking of Family Ties* (Routledge). She is currently clinical lead for a randomized controlled trial of MBT for children with emotional and behavioural difficulties, the ERiC study.

Nicole Muller is a child and adolescent psychotherapist and family therapist at Centrum Hecht in Holland, a specialist centre for the treatment of children, youth and their families, specialized in attachment and trauma problems. She is a MBT-CYP practitioner, supervisor, and trainer for Anna Freud London, and with her colleagues she runs Centrum Hecht Opleidingen in Holland, a training centre specialized in MBT-CYP. She has written many articles on MBT and is co-author of *Mentalization-Based Treatment for Children: A Time-Limited Approach* (APA, 2017/2026).

Momoko Nakanishi is a clinical psychologist and a certified public psychologist in Japan. She is also an MBT-C practitioner and supervisor certified by Anna Freud. Currently, she serves as a special lecturer at Konan University, where she trains aspiring certified public psychologists. She also works as a supervisor at child psychotherapy facilities and children's homes.

Maria Højer Nannestad is a consultant clinical psychologist specializing in children, adolescence and families who have lived with domestic violence. She is one of the founders of the NGO Institut mod vold (www.institutmodvold.dk) and the private practice Pyskologisk Perspektiv in Denmark (www.psykologiskperspektiv.dk), where she arranges 2-year-long MBT training courses. Maria offers mentalization-based treatment for traumatized children and adolescents in cooperation with different organizations, including Kvindehjemmet (a women's shelter), where she has groups for children after their stay at a shelter.

Marcia Olhaberry is a clinical psychologist, PhD in psychotherapy, and associate professor at the School of Psychology, Pontificia Universidad Católica de Chile. In 2023, she co-authored the book *Mentalization-Based Treatment for Children: Clinical Applications in the Current Context* (Herder). Her main research interests include early mental health prevention and intervention, perinatal depression, trauma, attachment, mentalization and parenting, as well as dyadic and triadic family interactions and bonds.

Sheila Redfern is a consultant clinical child and adolescent psychologist at Anna Freud, London, England, and director of Redfern Psychology. She has worked with children, adolescents, and their parents and caregivers in mental health settings for thirty years. She has presented on BBC Radio 4 Woman's Hour, Channel 5 news and is a regular contributor to BBC Bitesize, where she gives practical advice and support to children and young people on the everyday issues affecting them in their lives, including the impact of national and global events on their mental health and well-being. Her first book, *Reflective Parenting*, has been used by parents and professionals across the world.

Saara Salo is a clinical psychologist with PhD in developmental psychology, working as a senior researcher at the Helsinki University, Finland. She has worked for 20 years as a therapist, supervisor and trainer on early inter-action starting already prenatally. She is currently the head of two national clinical study projects on perinatal mentalizing- and play-based interven-tions among parents with substance-abuse disorder and/or mental health problems.

Miguel M. Terradas is a professor at the Department of Psychology, Uni-versité de Sherbrooke, Quebec, Canada. He is also a researcher at the Youth in Difficulty University Institute. He co-authored several articles concerning a mentalizing approach in youth protection services. As a clin-ician, he works with children suffering from the consequences of complex trauma living in foster care.

Hanneke van Aalst is a clinical psychologist and psychotherapist, specialized in MBT. She is the clinical head of the MBTC department where she and her team treat families with complex problems, at the Viersprong, Holland. She is also a MBT-supervisor and MBTtrainer.

Nicole Vliegen is a child and adolescent psychotherapist and a professor of clinical psychology at KU Leuven, Belgium. She heads the postgraduate training programmes in psychodynamic child psychotherapy and infant mental health, and the team of psychodynamic child psychotherapists at PraxisP, the clinical centre of KU Leuven. She co-authored *Therapeutic Work with Children with Complex Trauma: A Three Track Psychodynamic Approach* (Routledge).

Junko Yagi is a child psychiatrist and professor at Iwate Medical University Hospital in Japan and principal investigator of the Michinoku Children's Cohort, a longitudinal study of parent-child mental health after the Great East Japan Earthquake, and an Asian regional trainer for trauma-focused CBT. She is the head of the Children's Section of the PTSD Treatment Guidelines Committee of the Japanese Society for Traumatic Stress Studies.

Foreword

As the founder and director of the Cultivating Compassion Lab, a mentalization-based treatment initiative for children and families presenting with ADHD symptoms, I have been deeply influenced by the work that Nick Midgley and his colleagues have done, which has helped us to develop a treatment model aimed at improving relationships between children with ADHD and the significant individuals in their lives. Over the past five years, I have conducted extensive research, trained and supervised doctoral psychology candidates, authored articles, and delivered presentations on the application of mentalization in working with children and parents. Through these experiences, I have found the approach to be transformative for children and their relationships with their families. With over 25 years of experience as a clinical psychologist specializing in children and families, I can confidently say that the past five years have been among the most impactful, particularly in helping parents cultivate compassion for their children who present with challenging and, at times, seemingly intractable behaviours.

It was not until the late twentieth century that the concept of complex trauma began to gain traction. For the field of psychology and psychiatry, there was a marked shift in recognizing that trauma, such as chronic abuse or exposure to domestic violence, can have prolonged adverse psychological impacts distinct from those associated with a PTSD diagnosis. Later, in the early 2000s, researchers like van der Kolk and colleagues linked complex trauma to interpersonal trauma experienced during early life and argued for the need for tailored therapeutic approaches. Developmental trauma, a subset of complex trauma, refers explicitly to trauma occurring in early childhood, affecting critical developmental stages such as brain development, emotional regulation, attachment, and social functioning. One therapeutic approach that has shown success in addressing interpersonal trauma in adults is mentalization-based treatment. While many books have been written about applying mentalization-based therapy to school-aged children, there has been a growing need for a resource dedicated to how counsellors and therapists can work with traumatized children and their families using this approach. This book fills that gap, addressing the pressing need for practical guidance on employing mentalization-based treatment to help children and families impacted by developmental trauma.

Mentalization-based treatment (MBT) is particularly suited to addressing the interpersonal nature of complex trauma experienced by children. By focusing on the child's capacity to understand and reflect on their own and others' mental states, MBT provides a framework for rebuilding trust and fostering secure attachment relationships. This book goes beyond merely connecting the dots between developmental trauma in children and the role of mentalization. It also addresses a critical gap in the field of child treatment: the relevance of this approach to diverse populations. Much of the existing literature on either developmental trauma or mentalization-based treatment in children lacks representation from diverse cultural and socioeconomic backgrounds. However, this book emphasizes the application of mentalization-based treatment across various global populations, enhancing its generalizability. With contributions from experienced clinicians and researchers, including the originators of the MBT-C (Mentalization-Based Treatment for Children) model, this book stands as a valuable resource for practitioners worldwide. Its global reach, for example, featuring perspectives from the Netherlands, the United Kingdom, Canada, Spain, Turkey, and Japan, adds to its richness and relevance.

Throughout my clinical practice, I have worked with numerous children and families who have experienced disruptions in their attachment to primary caregivers. These disruptions often stem from chronic neglect, physical and emotional abuse, inconsistent caregiving, substance misuse and abuse, the loss of a parent, or institutionalized care following removal from the home. While the causes of these disruptions vary, the impact on the child's development often extends far beyond the immediate trauma, setting a psychological template for the individual's relational world that can have lasting consequences well into adulthood. Understanding how these early childhood experiences alter a child's developmental trajectory, with potentially enduring effects on their emotional, cognitive, and social functioning, makes the insights presented in this book even more compelling and vital.

The cases detailed in this book vividly capture the complexity of the interpersonal dynamics between children and their caregivers. Any therapist or parent reading these cases will resonate with the efforts of parents and children to connect amid significant challenges. For example, as I read the cases, I found myself relating deeply to the depiction of a child's seemingly unpredictable and dysregulated emotional life and the parent's struggle with conflicting emotions, from a desire to comfort their child to feelings of frustration and anger when their efforts seem to fall short. In my experience, adopting a mentalization framework allows therapists to appreciate the dialectical nature of the interactions: vulnerability and defensiveness, pleasure and anger, or effectiveness and futility. This perspective makes this challenging work more tolerable and fosters compassion for all parties involved. Most importantly, this approach has enabled me to witness profound transformations in the relationships between caregivers and their children.

The book is invaluable for clinicians working with children, parents, or both. It provides practical applications of the MBT-C approach to treating children and parents affected by developmental trauma. While each chapter can stand alone, readers who engage with the entirety of the book will gain a comprehensive understanding of the model, tools to enhance their clinical practice and efficacy of therapeutic outcomes. The multidimensional nature of the book, spanning topics from assessment to treatment, individual to systemic interventions, and a diverse global perspective, ensures that readers can find content relevant to their specific interests and professional needs.

One of the strengths of this book lies in its emphasis on integrating developmental science with clinical practice. The authors provide a detailed exploration of how early experiences of trauma and disrupted attachment shape the child's developmental trajectory, affecting their capacity for self-regulation, emotional expression, and interpersonal relationships. By grounding their approach in developmental research, the authors offer a solid theoretical foundation for clinicians seeking to understand the complex interplay between trauma, attachment, and mentalization. This integration of theory and practice makes the book both intellectually rigorous and clinically practical.

Another notable feature of this book is its commitment to inclusivity. The authors address a critical gap in the existing literature by highlighting the application of MBT-C across diverse cultural and socioeconomic contexts. Too often, therapeutic models are developed and validated within narrow populations, limiting their applicability to the broader, more diverse populations clinicians encounter. This book's global perspective, featuring case studies and research from various countries, demonstrates the adaptability and relevance of the MBT-C model to different cultural contexts. This inclusivity not only enhances the book's appeal, but also underscores the universality of mentalization as a therapeutic principle.

The book also offers practical tools and techniques for clinicians, including guidelines for assessment, intervention strategies, and case examples that illustrate the application of the MBT-C model in real-world settings. These tools are designed to help clinicians navigate the complexities of working with traumatized children and their families, providing concrete strategies for fostering mentalization and improving attachment relationships. For example, the authors provide detailed descriptions of how to use interventions to enhance the child's capacity for mentalization, as well as strategies for helping parents reflect on their mental states and those of their children. These practical insights make the book a valuable resource for both novice and experienced clinicians.

In addition to its clinical applications, the book also has implications for broader systems of care. By addressing the systemic factors that contribute to developmental trauma, such as socioeconomic inequality, family instability, and inadequate access to mental health services, the authors highlight the importance of adopting a holistic approach to treatment. This systemic perspective is particularly relevant for clinicians working in community-based settings, where the impact of these broader factors is often most acutely felt. By integrating individual, family, and systemic interventions, the MBT-C model provides a comprehensive framework for addressing the multifaceted challenges of developmental trauma.

The transformative potential of the MBT-C approach is best illustrated through the case studies included in the book. These cases provide vivid, real-life examples of how mentalization-based treatment can help children and their families overcome the challenges of developmental trauma. The authors detail the therapeutic process with clarity and sensitivity, capturing the nuances of the child's emotional world and the parent's journey toward greater understanding and empathy. These stories serve as powerful reminders of the resilience of the human spirit and the capacity for growth and healing, even in the face of significant adversity.

In conclusion, I highly recommend this book to clinicians working with children and families affected by developmental trauma. Its practical application of the MBT-C model and its theoretical depth and commitment to inclusivity make it an invaluable resource for practitioners seeking to enhance their clinical practice. Whether you are a seasoned clinician or new to the field, this book offers a wealth of insights and tools to support your work with traumatized children and their families. By engaging with the book's multidimensional approach, spanning assessment, treatment, and systemic interventions, readers will gain a deeper understanding of the complexities of developmental trauma and the transformative potential of mentalization-based treatment. Above all, this book serves as a testament to the power of compassion and understanding in fostering healing and connection in the lives of children and their families.

Francine Conway, PhD
Distinguished Professor, Graduate School of Applied and Professional Psychology, Rutgers University–New Brunswick

Introduction

A mentalization-based approach to working with children

Nicole Muller, Emma Morris and Nick Midgley

Up to a third of children growing up worldwide experience some type of childhood maltreatment (Stoltenborgh et al., 2015). Children who experience such maltreatment, especially from within their own families, can experience a wide range of psychological and physical consequences. As these children reach school age, they may find themselves being diagnosed with oppositional defiant disorder (ODD), attention deficit hyperactivity disorder (ADHD) or generalized anxiety, and be offered a range of different types of medication or psychological interventions. But too often these may leave the underlying impact of early maltreatment unattended to.

Our motivation in putting together this edited book is to bring together some of the creative ways in which practitioners are trying to respond to the needs of this group of children, drawing on a mentalization-based treatment (MBT) framework. MBT is an evidence-based treatment that was initially developed for adults with borderline personality disorders (Bateman & Fonagy, 2004). Mentalizing – the capacity to understand oneself and others in terms of intentional mental states such as needs, desires, feelings, beliefs, and goals – may be limited in those with borderline personality disorder. Enhancement of mentalization and improved emotional regulation are at the core of MBT treatment. Building on the principles of the original model of MBT for adults developed by Peter Fonagy and Antony Bateman, therapists from around the world who work with children, young people and families have developed adaptations of MBT for work with different age groups, and different clinical presentations (for overviews of the work with children, young people and families, see Midgley & Vrouva, 2012; Byrne et al., 2021; Midgley et al., 2021).

In recent years, one area of significant development has been in adaptations of MBT to address the specific needs of those who have experienced trauma. For adults, this has led to the creation of a specific "trauma-focused" model of MBT (Smits et al., 2024); while in the case of work with children, young people and families, it has led to a range of creative adaptations, responsive to the various different contexts in which help may be needed. Such adaptations are the focus of this book, which offers a series of case examples of mentalization-based work

DOI: 10.4324/9781032713441-1

with children, their families and the networks surrounding those children. As this work has been taking place in various parts of the world, and needs to be responsive to different cultural contexts, the chapters in this book draw on work by practitioners from a range of countries, including those in Western Europe, Scandinavia, North and South America, and Southeast Asia.

Chapter 1 provides an overview of the concept of developmental trauma itself and explores how it may impact on a child's development. Rather than providing a detailed overview of the psychological research in this field, it will focus – from a clinical perspective – on some of the ways in which a child who has experienced developmental trauma may present, and the implications of this for those aiming to provide psychological support.

The rest of the book is divided into three parts, each focusing on a different aspect of mentalization-based treatment for children who have experienced developmental trauma. In Part I, we look at the way in which a mentalizing lens can inform the assessment of children and their families, in the context of trauma. Nicole Vliegen and Norka Malberg (Chapter 2) provide a clinical account of how the assessment of children can be used as a basis for "scaffolding" treatment, while Karin Ensink and Jordan Bate (Chapter 3) give a perspective on the assessment of parents and carers.

In Part II of the book, we turn to explore the direct therapeutic work in time-limited MBT with school-age children who have experienced developmental trauma. Marcia Olhaberry (Chapter 4), from Chile, provides a detailed account of her work with a younger child, Isidora, 4 years old. This is followed Momoko Nakanishi and Junko Yagi (Chapter 5) providing a case study of the work with "Taro", a 9-year-child from Japan; Sibel Halfon, Hazal Çelik, and Dilara Güvenç (Chapter 6) describing work done with "Pamir", a 9-year-old child in Turkey; and Natasha Dobrova-Krol and Nicole Muller (Chapter 7) describing the work with "Yurko", a displaced Ukrainian boy, 8 years old, living in the Netherlands, due to the war in his country. These are followed by an account by Maria Højer Nannestad (Chapter 8), from Denmark, of how a mentalization-based group treatment can be creatively used to meet the needs of children, like Ingrid (10 years old) and Amir (12 years old) who have experienced domestic violence.

As therapists working with children know well, interventions with children always take place in a wider context, and the most effective therapies include a focus on carers, parents and the wider network surrounding each child. So in Part III of the book we turn our attention to the wider system, and how mentalization-based ideas can be creatively adapted for use in this type of work. We begin with a chapter by Saara Salo from Finland (Chapter 9), describing a mentalization-based approach to working with traumatized children and traumatized parents together. Chapter 10 is written by Masja Juffermans and Hanneke van Aalst, both from Holland, describing how mentalization-based work with parents – who have often experienced their own adverse childhood experiences – can go alongside child therapy, aiming to address issues related to "blocked care" in the parents themselves. This is followed in Chapter 11 by an important interview, conducted by Emma Morris, with C. Evans, the adoptive mother of a child who attended MBT, due to the complex impact of early trauma in her life. This interview provides a very powerful account of the "lived experience" of being the parent of a child who is living with the consequences of such adversity, as well as the experience of engaging in MBT from the perspective of a "service user".

We then have two chapters describing mentalization-based interventions with the wider network: Vincent Domon-Archambault and Miguel M. Terradas (Chapter 12) describe their work in Canada to engage with youth protection services; and Sheila Redfern and Nick Midgley from the UK (Chapter 13) describe the Reflective Fostering Programme, a group-based intervention for foster and kinship carers. In Chapter 14 a recapitulation of the clinical adaptations of the mentalization-based treatment model for children in the context of developmental trauma is described.

As the brief description of these chapters makes clear, in this edited book we have aimed to have an international perspective on MBT work with children, and have invited all of the authors to reflect on how the cultural context in which they were working shaped how their mentalization-based approach has evolved. As the title of this book makes clear, this is primarily a "case book" – in other words, we invited authors to not simply provide theoretical descriptions of their work, but rather to give detailed accounts of the actual work, to allow readers to see, hear and feel what the work is like. In order to keep the focus on the clinical material, chapter authors do not provide detailed explanations of specific concepts derived from mentalization-based theory and treatment, so for those who are not familiar with these concepts, we provide a brief glossary of terms at the end of the book (we would encourage those unfamiliar with MBT to also consider reading introductory works such as those by Sharp & Bevington, 2023, Fonagy and Bateman, 2024, or Midgley et al. 2025).

Children who have experienced developmental trauma can enter the world outside of their caregiving relationship less able to attend to the internal states of themselves and others, less able to regulate their emotions, less able to explicitly mentalize and less able to "take in" learning from the world around them. This "developmental delay" can further reduce their opportunities for learning as they struggle to make use of social and educational input that is pitched at their chronological age but beyond their developmental stage. Furthermore, the social, emotional and behavioural difficulties that children experience related to developmental trauma and latent vulnerability can, in themselves, lead to the child experiencing further relational harm. Even those in the child's network who have a robust and well-developed mentalizing capacity can experience the child as "difficult" and respond in non-mentalizing ways by disengaging or reacting in a punitive, hostile or controlling fashion, focusing on behaviour. This type of response heightens further the distress and anxiety in the child and can trigger even more "difficult" behaviour which is hard to mentalize and leads to an escalating cycle of non-mentalizing responses. As a result, the child who already experiences a difficulty in making relationships will experience further erosion of their social network, something that is referred to as "social thinning" (Van Harmelen et al., 2017).

Socio-cultural factors can impact on the way a system responds to a traumatized child. Bias and prejudice inherent in all societies and institutions, can impact on the meaning given to a child's behaviour and evaluation of a carer's response. For example, a professional such as a teacher or therapist may make different attributions about a violent child's motivations or intentions based on prejudice associated with factors such as the child's race, ethnicity, gender, faith or social class. Similarly, imposition of dominant cultural views about child-rearing can lead to the professional network being dismissive of carers potentially valid suggestions about how to understand and respond to a child. Finally, being blind to privilege can block professionals from seeing the impact of social factors such as oppression and poverty on a family's mentalizing capacity and foster a "blaming" culture. Consideration of social and cultural factors is of particular importance to therapists working with developmental trauma not just because socially disadvantaged and minor- itized families are over-represented in this group, but also due to the increased risk that the therapists mentalizing capacity can be thrown offline in response to trauma symptomology. It is in these moments that we are most likely to revert to sub-conscious bias, defend against cultural dis- comfort and guilt associated with privilege, and find it most difficult to adopt a culturally humble position.

While the parenting practices, interpretation of behaviour and affective responses of the families and therapists described in this book are heavily influenced by different social and cultural constructs, values and norms, the contributing authors are working towards a shared aim: To strengthen men- talizing in families, with the belief that this will lead to greater capacity for emotion regulation, for building a stronger sense of self and promoting sup- portive relationships and the capacity to engage in social learning. The emphasis on curiosity, uncertainty and non-judgement adopted by MBT practitioners, which sits well with a position of cultural humility, in addition to the focus on social learning allows for a level of cultural flexibility. In this sense it could be argued that MBT is not only a trans-diagnostic model, but also trans-cultural one. However, there are certain cultural limitations of the model that it is important to acknowledge. For example, research supporting attachment theory, which forms the theoretical foundation of MBT, is bias towards white western populations, and there is little known about the devel- opment of mentalizing across different cultures (Aival-Naveh et al., 2019).

Many of the basic principles of MBT can be applied in cases of develop- mental trauma. However, there are some adaptations which can be made with regard to focus, frame and pace. These are largely the focus of this book.

Through case examples, the nature of MBT practice with developmentally traumatized children and their families is illustrated.

Two final points on language and terminology. Firstly, throughout this book we will use the term carer and "parent" to refer to any adult that has a primary caregiving role in the child's life. This choice is because we view "parent" as a role that one can assume or play in a variety of ways. There is often more than one parent, whether there are two biological parents, adoptive parents, same-sex parents, step-parents, other family members playing a parenting role, or non-kinship carers (foster carers, other adults that provide caregiving on a continuous basis). Secondly, we have asked authors to use core terms related to mentalization-based treatment freely, without having to stop and explain or define what those terms mean. For readers who are familiar with MBT, we hope this will make your read smoother, and will reduce unnecessary repetition; readers who are less familiar with MBT (or would welcome a reminder) will find it useful to refer to the glossary at the end of the book.

References

Aival-Naveh, E., Rothschild-Yakar, L., & Kurman, J. (2019). Keeping culture in mind: A systematic review and initial conceptualization of mentalizing from a cross-cultural perspective. *Journal of Clinical Psychology* 26 (4). https://doi:10.1111/cpsp.12300.

Bateman, A. W., & Fonagy, P. (2004). *Psychotherapy for borderline personality disorder: Mentalization- based treatment.* Oxford University Press.

Byrne, G., Murphy, S., & Connon, G. (2020). Mentalization-based treatments with children and families: A systematic review of the literature. *Clinical Child Psychology and Psychiatry* 25 (4), 1022–1048. doi:10.1177/1359104520920689.

Fonagy, P. & Bateman, A. (2024). *Handbook of Mentalizing in Mental Health Practice,* 2nd edition. American Psychiatric Publications. doi:10.1176/appi.books.9781615379019.lg01.

Midgley, N. & Vrouva, I. (2012). *Mentalizing the child: Mentalization-Based Interventions with Children, Young People and their Families.* Routledge. doi:10.4324/9780203123003.

Midgley, N., Sprecher, E. A., & Sleed, M. (2021). Mentalization-based interventions for children aged 6–12 and their carers: A narrative systematic review. *Journal of Infant, Child, and Adolescent Psychotherapy,* 20 (2), 169–189. doi:10.1080/15289168.2021.1915654.

Midgley, N., Ensink, K., Lindqvist, K., Malberg, N., & Muller, N. (2025). *Mentalization-based treatment for children: A time-limited approach,* 2nd edition. American Psychological Association.

Sharp, C., & Bevington, D. (2023). *Mentalizing in psychotherapy: A guide for practitioners.* Routledge.

Smits, M. L., de Vos, J., Rüfenacht, E., Nijssens, L., Shaverin, L., Nolte, T., Luyten, P., Fonagy, P., & Bateman, A. (2024). Breaking the cycle with trauma-focused mentalization-based treatment: theory and practice of a trauma-focused group intervention. *Frontiers of Psychology* (15), 1–17. doi:10.3389/fpsyg.2024.1426092.

Stoltenborgh, M., Bakermans-Kranenburg, M., Alink, L., & Van IJzendoorn, M. (2015). The prevalence of child maltreatment across the globe: Review of a series of meta-analyses. *Child Abuse Review*, 24 (37–50). doi:10.1002/car.2353.

Van Harmelen, A. L., Kievit, R. A., Ioannidis, K., Neufeld, S., Jones, P. B., Bullmore, E., Dolan, R., NSPN Consortium, Fonagy P., & Goodyer I. (2017). Adolescent friendships predict later resilient functioning across psychosocial domains in a healthy community cohort. *Psychological Medicine* 47 (13), 2312–2322. doi:10.1017/S0033291717000836.

Part I

Introduction and theoretical overview

Chapter 1

The impact of developmental trauma on children

A mentalizing perspective

Nicole Muller and Emma Morris

What is developmental trauma?

Developmental or "complex" trauma refers to "the experience of multiple, chronic and prolonged, developmentally adverse traumatic events, most often of an interpersonal nature (e.g, sexual or physical abuse, war, community violence) and early-life onset" (van der Kolk, 2009). These experiences, which are also referred to as "relational" (Schore, 2013) or "attachment" (Allen, 2013) trauma, most often occur within the child's caregiving system and include physical, emotional, and educational neglect and child maltreatment beginning in early childhood. Although developmental trauma is often framed in terms of the parent–child relationship, and the failure of a carer to provide a safe and nurturing experience for a child, it is important to understand this within a broader perspective. Social and cultural resources, social integration and cohesiveness and community support can have a significant impact on a carer's capacity to provide a safe relational and developmental context for their child and contribute to the family's and child's wellbeing and sense of security (Ioannidis et al., 2020). A child's experience of care and safety is mediated by their social context and can be significantly impaired as a result of social injustice.

In this chapter, after providing a brief overview of the impact of developmental trauma on children, we explore how developmental trauma may impact in particular on a child's capacity for epistemic trust, and on the "building blocks" of the child's capacity to mentalize. We set out some of the implications this may have for how the child is "in the world"; and how the wider world (including school) may respond to the child. Finally, implications for treatment are discussed, including key considerations when adapting mentalization-based treatments (MBT) for use with traumatized children and their carers.

The impact of developmental trauma

Children who have experienced developmental trauma may or may not have been physically harmed or unsafe, however, all have repeatedly "experienced being left alone in the most difficult emotional situation" (Allen et al., 2008).

DOI: 10.4324/9781032713441-3

This means that there was no one to help them emotionally at that moment, to accompany them in their suffering, validating their emotional state, helping them to find words, to make sense of it and helping them to recover. This experience can generate toxic stress in a child's brain and body (Teicher et al., 2016). Traumatized children can be stuck in fear-mode as they grow up, being hypervigilant, and therefore easily overwhelmed, often feeling endangered even when safe. When this situation is chronic it can have a long-term impact on their brain development, as well as their physical well-being, including the functioning of their immune system (Malberg & Dangerfield, 2022).

Learning how to cope with adversity is an important part of healthy child development. When we are threatened, our bodies prepare us to respond: by increasing our heart rate, blood pressure, and stress hormones, such as cortisol or to hold still or play dead depending on the threat and relational context. When a young child's stress response systems are activated within an environment of supportive relationships with adults, these physiological effects are buffered and brought back down to baseline. The result is the development of healthy stress response systems. However, if the stress response is extreme and long-lasting, and buffering relationships are unavailable to the child, the result can be damaged, weakened systems and brain architecture, with lifelong repercussions. When a toxic stress response occurs continually, or is triggered by multiple sources, it can have a cumulative toll on an individual's physical and mental health. The more adverse experiences in childhood, the greater the likelihood of developmental delays and later health problems, including heart disease, diabetes, substance abuse, and depression (Danese et al., 2020).

Fear and threat detection not only shape an individual child's way of seeking safety and closeness but also their exploratory behaviour. The tendency to find comfort in others, discovering the world of people and things play a key role in our survival and ongoing development; it is how we come to make sense of the world around us. Optimally, fear is diminished by the attachment figure, grounding exploration in a feeling of safety, authenticity, and freedom. However, when carers have played a part in a child's traumatic experiences, not only are the carers not available as a "safe base" to help the child cope with these experiences, they themselves are connected with or the source of the traumatic experience. Children are dependent on their caregivers and they have to stick to them for survival. However, when their caregiver is also a source of threat, they have to simultaneously protect themselves from them and so they develop strategies to maintain the best level of care and safety they can in a precarious, unsafe relational context. This may include fight, flight or freeze responses, compartmentalisation and detachment, dissociation or avoidance of certain affect, sensations, thoughts and memories. These strategies are largely unconscious and automatic. They are primitive survival strategies, keeping the child who is totally dependent on the care of the abusive or neglectful adult, alive. However, while such strategies can be effective in maintaining the best care available to a child, they often come at great cost when it comes to a child's functioning outside of the neglectful or abusive caregiving relationship and their developmental trajectory more generally (Vliegen et al., 2023a, 2023b).

McCrory and Viding (2015) use the term "latent vulnerability" to describe the way that such early adaptations among maltreated children are associated with cognitive and neurological differences which make these children vulnerable to the development of social, emotional and behavioural difficulties later on. For example, differences have been observed among children from maltreated populations in the way that they process threatening information, in that they are more vigilant and over sensitive to threat cues. While such strategies may be adaptive in an abusive or neglectful caregiving relationship, this processing style can be maladaptive in a school context, leading these children to overreact or use avoidance strategies in the face of perceived threat. Allocation of attentional and cognitive resources to potential threat cues can lead them to miss other potentially helpful information in their internal or external environment. Children who have experienced developmental trauma are also less likely to recognise or respond to rewards due to the experience of receiving care in which positive feedback was absent, inconsistent or incongruent. In this context, the child either doesn't recognise rewards in the first instance, or protects themselves from disappointment by not attending to it. However, in more everyday contexts it is likely to be associated with anhedonia, reduced motivation to engage in developmentally supportive interaction or activity and reduced opportunities for positive self-affirmation.

Thus, latent vulnerability increases the risk that social, emotional and behavioural difficulties will develop in a child in the sense that they can block the child's engagement with opportunities to grow and learn from the world around them. When in survival mode, even small changes, like altered routines, moving from one classroom to another, new situations, slightly raised voices, can signal "life or death danger" and automatically trigger, what is in the child's mind and body, a disproportionate response. All the child's resources are "employed" and focused on staying alive physically and staying in the minds of their significant adults. This takes away their focus from processing and retaining new information and adversely further affects the development of emotion regulation academic and social learning, empathy and turn taking.

Developmental trauma and epistemic trust

It is important for every child, as they grow up, to discern not just who is to be trusted and who is benevolent and reliable as a source of information, but also who is uninformed, unreliable, or downright bad-intentioned. Being excessively open to trusting others is maladaptive, just as being excessively closed to the possibility of receiving relevant new information is maladaptive (Sperber et al., 2010; Wilson & Sperber, 2012). Traumatised individuals, carers and children, often protect themselves by shielding themselves from potentially harmful information and experiences (Knox, 2016). This can lead to what is termed epistemic vigilance or mistrust. Children can become closed to the social communication of knowledge that is crucial for their development. Avoidantly attached children and carers will often close themselves off: epistemic mistrust. Those with anxious-ambivalent attachment often rely too heavily on one attachment figure and have developed too little autonomy, to suspend that trust when necessary. That makes them vulnerable to entanglement in dependent relationships. They are epistemically hypervigilant towards almost everyone, but epistemically naive towards that one attachment figure who knows how to reach them. (Hutsebaut, Nijssen, & Vessem 2023).

If a child's attachment figure is a source of both fear and trust, which is the case in disorganized attachment, the child often feels deeply confused and isolated. They dare not trust themselves or others. They will seek assurance from others but feel doubtful at the same time, engaging in a restless, if not obsessive, preoccupation with reading contextual cues (Fonagy & Allison, 2014; Fonagy, Luyten, & Allison, 2015). Due to epistemic hypervigilance and mistrust, the capacity to meet with other minds is often blocked when a child has experienced developmental trauma (Fonagy, Campbell, & Luyten, 2023).

Developmental trauma and the building blocks of mentalizing

In an earlier work (Midgley et al., 2017), we described how a child's development can be understood in terms of the "building blocks" of mentalizing – more specifically, the development of attention control, affect regulation and explicit mentalization. Whereas the adult model of MBT mostly focuses on the duality of mentalizing/non-mentalizing (or pre-mentalizing), we believe that work with children requires more of a developmental perspective, whereby "explicit mentalizing" is the top of a triangle, but that a child's capacity for explicit mentalization builds on (and then in turn supports) the more basic processes of attention control and affect regulation.

Midgley et al. (2017) suggest that this provides a useful conceptual framework when thinking about the clinical challenges of working with children who present with a range of emotional and/or behavioural problems, and how to address them in MBT. Here we briefly introduce these concepts and explore how developmental trauma may impact on each "level" of these building blocks.

Attention control

A baby develops by integrating bodily sensations and body awareness. Before a child is able to connect with themselves and others, they must first connect with their body. Babies initially learn about their bodies and the world around them through their senses. The ear catches sound and the eye notices light.

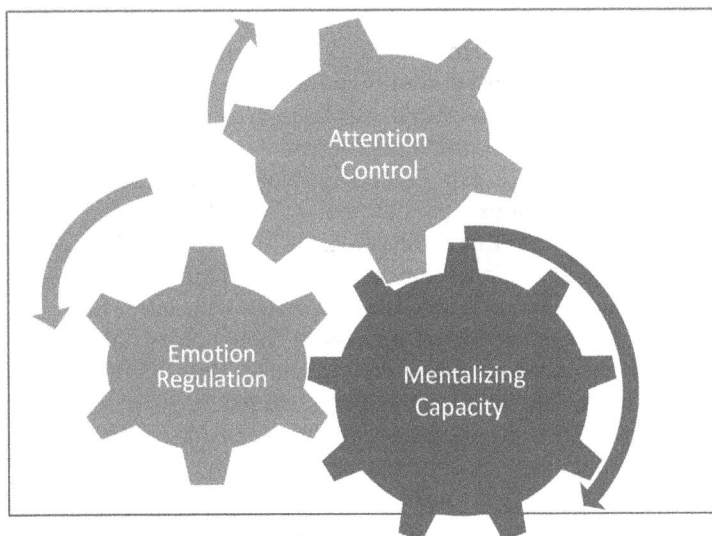

Figure 1.1 Building blocks of mentalizing.

They perceive pressure differences through their sense of touch, the tongue tastes and the nose smells. Each baby and each caregiver have their own style of moving. Sensory integration occurs when stimuli can be distinguished, and connections can be made. The child responds with the body. If a carer connects with a child, they can learn about body boundaries and body sensations. By literally holding them in a loving embrace (Winnicott, 1965), by being physically present and through touch, the carer can provide a secure attachment experience, attuned to the child. Touch used in a good way, can provide comfort, relieve pain, offer boundaries and stimulate children to explore and develop.

'Parental embodied mentalizing' is a carer's ability to implicitly recognise and understand a child's preferences, wishes and desires by paying attention to their physical expression and adapting accordingly with their own body (Shai & Fonagy, 2014). An attuned carer tries to imagine what is going on in the child and will try to mirror their feeling in a contingent and "marked" way; that is the carer provides a response that enables the child to connect with their experience and makes it clear to them that the emotion being mirrored by the carer is the baby's emotion and not the carer's emotion. This mirroring occurs partly implicitly, for example through the carer's body language, the sounds they make, the intonation of their voice and partly explicitly through the words expressed, based on the carer's reflections on the child and the interaction between them (Jensen et al., 2021). Sensory integration begins through this process in infancy but continues through childhood. Beliefs about self, others and the world, often formed in the interaction with carers, influence the posture, structure, and movements of the body and the mind. How a child is physically cared for, touched, experienced, loved or unloved, and how the other person perceives, reflects and mirrors the child, offers boundaries to them and provides a foundation for sensory integration and attention control.

For children who have experienced developmental trauma, bodily and sensory awareness develops very differently. When a child has been persistently abused or neglected by their caregiver, they have not had their states mirrored, or they have had them mirrored inaccurately. Some may have experienced overwhelming physical pain. All will have been left with overwhelming feelings of fear or distress in their bodies. Often this begins before a child has developed language to make sense of their experiences. All these memories are sensory memories, stored in their sensory system, unavailable for explicit recall. These children can have sensory flashbacks which means that they re-experience the bodily feeling of immediate danger, with no means to make sense of it or communicate about it. Often, they have not learned how to live and feel relaxed in their bodies because of the persistent stress or threat in the caregiving relationship, and so the connection between body, self-awareness and environment cannot be made. The disconnection between external reality, bodily experiences and mental states can be seen as an extreme form of pretend mode that serves a protective function (Muller & Midgley, 2017). Such disconnection allows the child to put unbearable feelings into different compartments. Dissociation can emerge as a survival response to trauma. It can serve as an unconscious defensive role by inhibiting children from connecting with their own pain, fear or shame and/ or the mental state of abusive caregivers (Allen, 2013), allowing them to escape in their mind when protection and care is unavailable. If a child has been abused and is then able to tell someone who does not believe the child, i.e. if there is double betrayal, the chance of developing dissociation and or amnesia is 67% (Wager, 2013) It can lead to a range of behaviours which can be misunderstood, such as daydreaming, withdrawal, lying, problems with concentration and behaviour (Struik, 2019).

Children who have experienced developmental trauma continually have their attention jolted and directed by the trauma that is carried within them and the strategies they have developed to protect themselves from this trauma and have no conscious control over this process. Trauma draws their attention outwards, it sharpens the senses and draws attention away from bodily signals. This happens at the time of the trauma, but also persists due to hypervigilance. Not paying attention to inside feelings and sensations is therefore not only avoidance, or due to dissociation, but also a consequence of hypervigilance. The opportunity to develop attentional control necessary for the development of emotional regulation and explicit mentalizing is vastly reduced in this context.

Emotion regulation

In a safe environment a child learns to recognise their own emotions through others. They learn to perceive their own signals and also those in the person nearby. The child experiences emotional arousal from physical signals and action patterns. In interaction with others, the child learns to assign words to physical sensations and to link them to emotions and their environment. Over time they gain an understanding of the internal and external contexts that give rise to particular affective states and how these can be regulated.

Children who experienced a carer–child relationship characterized by neglect or abuse have less opportunity to learn to recognize and regulate emotions. Children left with overwhelming and unfathomable affects often cannot assimilate these experiences in order to shape a sense of who they are in the world and in relation to others. Instead, they can learn that such states should be avoided at all costs. When a carer is unable to tune in to their child's inner state it can be incorrectly mirrored. For example, if a child is consistently responded to by being hit, shaken, ignored, mocked or met with parental fear or panic, they learn that their feelings are dangerous, that their feeling will hurt others or will hurt themselves. Great confusion can arise within the child about what they feel and to whom that feeling belongs. If a carer gets scared or angry because the child is uncomfortable, what is mirrored to, seen or experienced by the child from the carer is the other person's fear or anger, which does not match what is being experienced in their own body. The experience that the child will then store within itself is "if I don't feel comfortable, the person who cares for me and whom I need becomes afraid or angry with me". They learn to think that if they experience a powerful feeling, they will generate fear or anger in the other person, and so avoid or disconnect from such feelings rather than seeking care. Without the opportunity to learn how to recognize, predict, and regulate strong emotions, the child will continue to actively avoid such feelings.

Active avoidance of strong and distressing affect is unsustainable as a long-term strategy and eventually the child will become dysregulated in a way that is likely to be experienced as incongruent, confusing, controlling or disproportionate by themselves and those around them. They may cry, shout, explode, withdraw, stiffen, or, more often, turn quiet (Ensink et al., 2016a, 2016b). Young children who have experienced developmental trauma sometimes use self-stimulatory or self-destructive behaviours for relief, such as tearing their eyelashes out, banging their head against a wall, accident prone behaviours, or excessive masturbation. At the core of trauma experiences is a loss of control, feeling powerless or helpless. Acting in a self-stimulatory or self-destructive way can be a teleological means of gaining a sense of control. It is a way of regulating the physical and emotional arousal in a more tolerable and bearable way.

In summary, the capacity for emotional regulation can be impacted by developmental trauma in a number of ways; it can mean that children have less opportunity to learn to accurately identify and regulate affective states in themselves and others via contingent, marked mirroring, they can learn to actively avoid affective states that they are unable to understand or regulate, they can experience strong unprocessed sensations, memories and affect triggered by trauma stimuli, and they can experience high levels of shame. As a result, strong affects can feel fragmented, unpredictable and overwhelming. They just "happen" to the child and as such are expressed in ways that can be hard to understand, further reducing mentalizing capacity for all involved.

Explicit mentalizing

Explicit mentalizing refers to the capacity to consciously reflect and being able to verbally name and speak about mental states such as emotions, thoughts and intentions in relation to the self and others. Neuroscientists suggest that this capacity is subserved by newer brain circuits, which are more linked with symbolic and linguistic processing (Luyten & Fonagy, 2015). Tasks involving reasoning, effortful control and perspective-taking may be slower than the more automatic modes of mentalizing, but they make it possible for us to more carefully and deliberately make attributions about the emotions, thoughts and feelings of self and others. This allows us to consider whether our immediate reactions are actually warranted after we have considered the situation and then we can over-ride or adjust our first impressions to be in line with these reflections. We often make use of more controlled or explicit mentalizing when there has been a difficult situation, which demands some kind of active reflection to help make sense of it (Midgley et al., 2017).

The window of tolerance is the optimal arousal zone within which affect can be processed and explicit connections made. This is less "wide" for children who have experienced developmental trauma. Easily triggered trauma memories and feelings of shame and low self-worth all mean that arousal and affect is commonly too high or too low (for example with active avoidance or disassociation) for explicit mentalizing to take place; there is little space for reflection on "What is this about? Why am I feeling this? Why am I thinking this?", and thus for thoughts, feelings and affects to be mentalized.

With repeated exposure to unsafe or unreliable care the child learns not to seek comfort, protection and social engagement and the capacity for recovery is increasingly undermined and the "window" gets smaller.

The capacity to explicitly mentalize about one's own thoughts and feelings is an essential part of managing relationships, and modulating one's own emotional responses. An experience of consistently unsafe, poorly-attuned care or secrets in the family can disrupt a child's development of a stable self-concept, sense of agency and coherent autobiographical narrative. When asked to describe themselves, traumatized children might respond in a bizarre and disorganized way, or with active avoidance of mentalization through aggressive refusal to mentalize or silly and clownish behaviour. Trying to understanding what underlies these responses, and whether they can be adequately explained by cognitive immaturity, or are triggered by anxiety or trauma is a necessary component of the assessment.

Many children who have experienced abuse or neglect develop a deep sense of being to blame, "bad" or "unwanted" and this can become their template for how they see themselves and how they think others see them. Intense feelings of shame reflect a sense of negative evaluation by another person who is experienced as more powerful, leading to strong feelings of anger, helplessness, and inferiority (Goss et al., 1994) which in themselves are likely to impair mentalizing capacity. Children in this situation can have difficulty looking in the mirror and seeing themselves. They can also have difficulty looking at others, afraid of what they can expect. They often don't feel they belong and so go in search for validation which can make them vulnerable to being exploited. Reminders of traumatic events can trigger sensations, emotions and memories that have not been processed and integrated. This means that feelings or sensations linked to the event can feel as real as if they are happening again. As a result, these children often fall into a state of psychic equivalence, not able to distinguish between the real world and what they experience. Their body reacts with either too much or too little activation. Too much consists of an overall state of readiness in the body, ready to fight or run. Too little activation of the body produces numbness and paralysis, unresponsiveness, not noticing what is happening in the body, breaking down actions and emotional experience; a freeze or collapse response. Because children who have experienced developmental trauma spend so much time outside of the "zone of tolerance" they have less opportunity to develop the capacity to mentalize explicitly.

Factors influencing the impact of developmental trauma

Developmental trauma does not affect all children in the same way, and there are many risk and protective factors that can influence the impact of trauma in the context of the developing capacity to mentalize. These include how old the child was when they experienced the trauma, how often or how long they were exposed to the trauma for, who was involved, where the trauma took place and whether there was someone or a network of people who provided a protective shield for the child in the form of corrective or reparative experiences (*Angels in the Nursery*; Lieberman et al., 2005). Resilience factors such as the child's overall functioning and their personality style or temperament can also mitigate the impact of trauma, as can the broader social, cultural and economic factors, such as privilege, poverty and discrimination.

Sometimes a child who has experienced developmental trauma may also have experienced other trauma outside of the caregiving relationship. They may have experienced impersonal or interpersonal trauma, such as war or displacement (described in Chapter 7) or secondary trauma, such as being exposed to another family member's traumatic experience in some way, as is often true for foster or adoptive carers who come to hear about the abuse and neglect their child experienced prior to being adopted, (described in Chapters 11 and 13). Or they may have experienced traumatic bereavement, such as the sudden death, suicide or homicide of a family member under circumstances that mean the child is unable to process the loss. Or the child may have experienced intergenerational trauma, such as living in a culture that carries a history of trauma or being cared for by a parent who has also experienced abuse or neglect as a child (described in Chapter 5).

In attachment theory a premise is that attachment style can be transmitted from one generation to the next. With respect to trauma this means that unresolved trauma in a carer may impact their capacity to respond sensitively to their child to the extent that the carer (often non-consciously) reproduces the disorienting and/or frightening behaviour that they themselves experienced (Fonagy et al., 2023). As a result the parents attachment trauma is revisited to the child, described by Fraiberg et al. (1975) as "ghosts in the nursery". The cycle can rapidly become malign. The carer's temporary emotional unavailability can generate further powerful distress in the child, which, when it resonates with the carer's own experience, can have the effect of further increasing the carer's arousal. The carer may re-experience their own childhood helplessness, now visibly displayed in the child:

> The escalating non-mentalizing interchanges may include violence as the 'solution' to terminate a deeply disturbing cycle. The carer's scream for the child to stop is a 'cry in the wilderness' to an emotionally dysregulated young brain. Unable to inhibit distress or put feelings into words, the child's response is likely to be physical. This can take the form of violence against others or the self, creating illusion of communication; it generates a reaction, but not one that necessarily matches the internal experience that is driving the child's actions.
>
> (Asen & Fonagy, 2017, p. 14)

Research about mentalizing capacity in traumatized parents shows us that family members are less likely to look at, or pay attention towards each other, to make physical contact to recognise emotions in themselves or their child and there are often trauma triggers in the behaviour of the child that triggers the parent. Traumatised parents can find it more difficult to provide (physical) comfort and demonstrate less tolerance of their children's distress. In these families there are often less discussions or moments to share ideas about emotions or different perspectives on social interactions, less mentalizing about their child, low parental reflective functioning (misattributions) and fewer opportunities for rupture and repair (Ensink et al., 2014, 2016a; Rutherford, 2015).

References

Allen, J. G. (2013). *Mentalizing in the development and treatment of attachment trauma.* Karnac Publishers.

Allen, J. G., Fonagy, P., & Bateman, A. W. (2008). *Mentalizing in clinical practice.* American Psychiatric Publishing.

Asen, E. & Fonagy, P. (2017). Mentalizing family violence part 1: Conceptual framework. *Family Process,* 56 (1), 6–21. doi:10.1111/famp.12261.

Danese, A., McLaughlin, K. A., Samara, M., & Stover, C. S. (2020). Psychopathology in children exposed to trauma: detection and intervention needed to reduce downstream burden. *British Medical Journal,* (19), 371–3073. doi:10.1136/bmj.m3073.

Ensink, K., Berthelot, N., Bernazzani, O., Normandin, L., & Fonagy, P. (2014). Another step closer to measuring the ghosts in the nursery: Preliminary validation of the Trauma Reflective Functioning Scale. *Frontiers of Psychology,* 17 (5), 1471. doi:10.3389/fpsyg.2014.01471.

Ensink, K., Bégin, M., Godbout, L., Normandin, N., & Fonagy, P. (2016a). Mentalization and dissociation in the context of trauma: Implications for child psychopathology. *Journal of Trauma Dissociation,* 18 (1), 11–30. doi:10.1080/15299732.2016.1172536.

Ensink, K., Normandin, L., Plamondon, A., Berthelot, N., & Fonagy, P. (2016b). Intergenerational pathways from reflective functioning to infant attachment through parenting. *Canadian Journal of Behavioural Science/Revue canadienne des sciences du comportement,* 48 (1), 9–18. doi:10.1037/cbs0000030.

Fonagy, P., Campbell, C., & Luyten, P. (2023). Attachment, mentalizing and trauma: Then (1992) and Now (2022). *Brain Science,* 13, 459. doi:10.3390/brainsci13030459.

Fonagy, P. & Allison, E. (2014). The role of mentalizing and epistemic trust in the therapeutic relationship. *Psychotherapy,* 51 (3), 372–380. doi:10.1037/a0036505.

Fonagy, P., Luyten, P., & Allison, E. (2015). Epistemic petrification and the restoration of epistemic trust: A new conceptualization of borderline personality disorder and its psychosocial treatment. *Journal of Personality Disorders* 29 (5), 575–609 doi:10.1521/pedi.2015.29.5.575.

Fonagy, P., Campbell, C., & Luyten, P. (2023). Attachment, mentalizing and trauma: Then (1992) and now (2022). *Brain Science,* 3 (3), 459. doi:10.3390/brainsci13030459.

Fraiberg, S., Adelson, E., & Shapiro, V. (1975). Ghosts in the nursery: A psychoanalytic approach to the problems of impaired infant-mother relationships. *Journal of the American Academy of Child Psychiatry* 14 (3), 387–421. doi:10.1016/S0002-7138(09)61442-61444.

Goss, K., Gilbert, P., & Allan, S. (1994). An exploration of shame measures: I. The Other As Shamer Scale. *Personality and Individual Differences,* 17 (5), 713–717. doi:10.1016/0191-8869(94)90149-X.

Hutsebaut, J., Nijssen, L., & Vessem, M. (2023). *The power of mentalizing: An introductory guide on mentalizing, attachment, and epistemic trust for mental health care workers.* Oxford Academic. doi:10.1093/oso/9780198880677.001.0001.

Ioannidis, K., Askelund, A. D., Kievit, R., & Van Harmelen, A. L. (2020). The complex neurobiology of resilient functioning after childhood maltreatment. *British Medical Journal,* 18 (1), 32. doi:10.1186/s12916-12020-1490-1497.

Jensen, T. J., Steen Høgenhaug, S., Kjølbye, M., & Skaalum Bloch, M. (2021). Mentalizing Bodies: Explicit mentalizing without words in psychotherapy. *Frontiers of Psychology,* 12, 577702. doi:10.3389/fpsyg.2021.577702.

Lieberman, A., Padrón, E., Van Horn, P., & Harris, W. W. (2005). Angels in the nursery: The intergenerational transmission of benevolent parental influences. *Journal of Infant Mental Health*, 26 (6), 504–520. doi:10.1002/imhj.20071.

Luyten, P. & Fonagy, P. (2015).The neurobiology of mentalizing. *Personal Disorders*. 6 (4): 366–379. doi:10.1037/per0000117.

Malberg, N. & Dangerfield, M. (2022). Young Kids: The impact of early adverse relational experiences. In Marsh, A. N. and Cox, L. J. (eds), *Not just bad kids: The adversity and disruptive behavior link* (pp. 311–320). Academic Press.

McCrory, E. J. & Viding, E. (2015). The theory of latent vulnerability: Reconceptualizing the link between childhood maltreatment and psychiatric disorder. *Development and Psychopathology*, 27 (2), 493–505. doi:10.1017/S0954579415000115.

Midgley, N., Ensink, K., Lindqvist, K., Malberg, N., & Muller, N. (2017). *Mentalization-based treatment for children: a time-limited approach*. American Psychiatric Association Publishing.

Muller, N. & Midgley, N. (2017). The clinical challenge of mentalization-based therapy with children who are in "pretend mode". *Journal of Infant, Child, and Adolescent Psychotherapy*, 19 (1). doi:10.1080/15289168.2019.1701865.

Rutherford, T. (2015). Emotional well-being and discrepancies between child and parent educational expectations and aspirations in middle and high school. *International Journal of Adolescence and Youth*, 20(1), 69–85. doi:10.1080/02673843.2013.767742.

Schore, A. N. (2013). Relational trauma, brain development, and dissociation. In J. D. Ford & C. A. Courtois (eds), *Treating complex traumatic stress disorders in children and adolescents: Scientific foundations and therapeutic models* (pp. 3–23). Guilford Press.

Shai, D. & Fonagy, P. (2014). Beyond words: Parental embodied mentalizing and the parent-infant dance. In M. Mikulincer & P. R. Shaver (eds), *Mechanisms of social connection: From brain to group* (pp. 185–203). American Psychological Association. doi:10.1037/14250-011.

Sperber D., Clément, H., Heintz, C., Mascaro, O., Mercier, H., Origgi, G., & Wilson, D. (2010). Epistemic Vigilance. *Mind & Language*, 25 (4), 359–393. doi:10.1111/j.1468-0017.2010.01394.x.

Struik, A. (2019). *Treating chronically traumatized children: The sleeping dogs method*, 2nd edition. Routledge. doi:10.4324/9780429021619.

Teicher, M. H., Samson, J. A., Anderson, C. M., & Ohashi, K. (2016).The effects of childhood maltreatment on brain structure, function and connectivity. *Nat Rev Neurosci.*, 17 (10), 652–666. doi:10.1038/nrn.2016.111.

van der Kolk, B. A., Pynoos, R. S., Cicchetti, D., Cloitre, M., D'Andrea, W., Ford, J. D., & Teicher, M. (2009). Proposal to include a developmental trauma disorder diagnosis for children and adolescents in DSM-V. www.cathymalchiodi. com/dtd_nctsn.pdf

Vliegen, N., Tang, E., & Meurs, P. (2023a) *Children recovering from complex trauma: From wound to scar*. Routledge.

Vliegen, N., Tang, E., Midgley, N., Luyten, P., & Fonagy, P. (2023b). *Therapeutic work for children with complex trauma: A three-track psychodynamic approach*. Routledge.

Wager, N. (2013). A scoping review considering the applicability of restorative justice to cases of sexual assault. International Psychological Applications Conference and Trends, Madrid, Spain.

Wilson, D. & Sperber, D. (2012). *Meaning and relevance*. Cambridge University Press.

Winnicott, D. W. (1965). *The maturational processes and the facilitating environment: Studies in the theory of emotional development*. International Universities Press.

Part II

The assessment of children who have experienced developmental trauma

Chapter 2

Drawing the picture

The assessment of children as scaffolding for treatment in the context of developmental trauma

Nicole Vliegen and Norka Malberg

"Although he is 7 years old, he displays quite a lot of toddler-like behaviour", the foster parents sigh at their first appointment at a child and adolescent mental health clinic in Belgium. Michael can over-react with anger for any little reason, he can't tolerate a no or a limit, bedtimes are hard times … His foster parents summarize the most difficult aspect of their relationship with Michael, his "unpredictability", which makes taking care of him and comforting him in difficult moments "suffocating". He is described as needing to be in motion constantly, particularly when distressed. The foster parents ask for help in understanding how Michael is thinking and feeling. They also want to understand what has been described as his "disappearing" in class and ask for help in providing him with the best family and social circumstances for growth and development.

Like many caregivers, Michael's foster parents seem confused and somewhat helpless. These feelings can prove to be quite contagious and at times lead to pre-mentalizing ways of functioning in parents, teachers and psychotherapists working with children who have experienced developmental trauma. In this chapter, we will describe the process of assessment as part of a referral for therapy and how it can potentially prove to be an opportunity to mentalize the child and their context. We will present the case of Michael[1] to illustrate the importance of considering assessment as an integral part of the treatment process in mentalization-based treatment with children (MBT-C; Midgley et al., 2017). Most importantly, this chapter seeks to highlight how the assessment period lends itself to laying the foundations for the development of epistemic trust with the child and their family. In MBT-C, this is achieved through the co-construction of a case formulation which will guide all involved during times of doubt and stress.

Getting started: assessment when the therapist is aware of developmental trauma

Children like Michael often present with diverse and complex symptoms. Learning about his problems in several areas and knowing he is a foster child, means that there is at least a possibility of developmental trauma in his

DOI: 10.4324/9781032713441-5

history. However, we never want to jump to conclusions as not every fostered child with mental health problems is a child who has experienced developmental trauma. To understand more about the child's presentation and to lay the foundations for epistemic trust, we begin with meeting the foster parents (hereafter referred to as "parents"). These sessions serve multiple purposes simultaneously:

a   Listening to the stories of these parents, looking at them together from a relational and developmental lens.
b   Getting an idea about the quality of relationships in the child's first years of life.
c   Getting to know the parents and listening for potential "ghosts in the nursery".
d   Validating and mentalizing the parents, developing a "we-mode".
e   Assessing parents' mentalizing capacity and the places where they are vulnerable to a mentalizing breakdown.
f   Considering what kind of individual assessment might be needed for the child.

Listening to the stories of parents

In the first meetings with parents, we listen to the content of their personal narratives and try to make sense of the difficulties they bring. Furthermore, we consider the quality of the interactions between the parents and the clinician, as important in order to set the framework when offering time-limited MBT for children (Midgley et al., 2017). What characterizes the emotional and relational functioning of a child with developmental trauma, is the fact that functioning is impacted in several domains. Therefore, we listen to the stories parents tell us, considering that developmentally traumatic experiences can influence the nature of a child's overall emotional and behavioural functioning. More specifically, such experiences can:

a   Interfere with the development of basic executive functioning and learning capacities, including capacities for stress regulation, attention, and focus.
b   Leave the child with particularly difficult affects and emotions and hinder the capacity to develop mature affect regulation and coping strategies.
c   Restrict the child's capacity to represent aspects of an inner world through play and to reflect on experiences.
d   Tax the development of secure relational skills and attachment representations.

In these first meetings, both parents described how Michael returned home after a school day dysregulated and stressed. He often seemed dissociated and presented with difficulties regarding executive functioning, specifically attentional control. Regarding affective development and affect regulation, there were difficulties in verbalization of emotions alongside high levels of physical dysregulation. He would move quickly from one thing to the next, empty out his toys and jump on the sofa "like a hurricane". The therapist wondered how his affective world looked, and what regulating and coping skills he had available. Michael's parents didn't seem to mention much about him thinking, feeling and expressing aspects of an inner world. As a result, the therapist wondered about the foster parents' reflective functioning capacities, that is their capacity to link their own and Michael's behaviours to mental states. There seemed to be a certain level of ambivalence manifested by Michael's foster parents regarding their willingness to step into Michael's world. The therapist wondered about the link between such ambivalence and what was described as Michael's "push and pull" behaviour towards his parents. What was his sense of safety?

Quality of relationships in the child's first years of life

During the first assessment session, Michael's current developmental issues and mental health needs were charted considering historical and contextual aspects of the child's specific developmental and relational story. While developmental trauma is a response to early adverse experiences, we need to picture the adverse experiences as well as possible because the child's early history can help us understand where the child needs to be met in terms of his current ways of functioning and the potential for development of epistemic trust.

During the second part of this initial session, his foster parents talked about Michael's start in life as characterized by unpredictability and neglect due to the harsh circumstances his birth parents were in, as chronic substance abusers. His biological mother – who had positive experiences with being fostered herself – chose voluntarily to put Michael up for foster care when he was a young toddler. His biological father died shortly after his birth from an overdose. Some years later, there was an attempt to reunite Michael and his mother, but the visits went badly. Michael reacted with intense separation anxiety from his foster parents, and his biological mother lacked the capacity to comfort him. When Michael's mother fell back into difficulties financially the family court decided he would stay on a more permanent basis with his foster family, and a fortnightly visit was established with her. Michael's experiences during his first years of life indicated the possibility of some of his difficulties being the result of developmental trauma, including the development of epistemic hypervigilance as an adaptive way of dealing with the unpredictability of his early relational environment.

Getting to know the foster family

Michael's foster parents were highly educated, professional people. They were both convinced there was room in their house and their lives to take care of a child who needed a family. Mother grew up in a warm family with a biological and a foster sister and felt this to be a positive experience. Father saw the positive aspects of this kind of parenting and easily accepted the idea of raising a foster child. Both parents were of a similar cultural and racial identity as Michael.

Of major importance to a family's ability to manage a vulnerable child's developmental and behavioural difficulties is the social support which the family can rely on. Therefore, as part of every assessment we also invite parents to talk about important "partners" in raising this child, and what kind of support or assistance these partners offer. Both maternal and paternal grandparents endorsed the idea of foster care and provided the family with practical and emotional support. Additionally, both parents had a good relationship with Max, a foster care worker who was strongly committed. Max actively supported the parents in their choice to ask for psychotherapeutic help.

Michael's parents spontaneously talked about how they found the period of reunification between Michael and his biological mother extremely stressful. To add to the stress of having to mourn the possible loss of Michael, the foster mother became pregnant and gave birth to twin boys. We wondered about the ambivalent feelings for these two parents regarding the process of supporting Michael and mentalizing his difficulties whilst going through the developmental process of being pregnant and having their own biological children. Furthermore, we were also curious about the impact of the birth of two birth children on Michael and the potential fear of losing his foster parents, which might relate to his separation anxiety.

Validating and mentalizing the parents

During the first meetings in any assessment, we listen to the parents' narratives about the difficulties they face and to the emotional impact these problems have on them and try to assess the family's current emotional atmosphere. We also observe the parents' capacity to develop a relationship with the clinician and their willingness to be open to social learning. In the work with Michael and his foster family, the therapist was impressed by the warmth and concern Michael's parents expressed when talking about their family, and about Michael. They seemed to express a longing to understand Michael better, a genuine curiosity which is an essential element of parental mentalizing. Their open request for help and support indicated the possibility of developing epistemic trust and their openness towards new social learning.

During the assessment it is important to mentalize the parents before we ask them to mentalize their child. For Michael's parents, it was highly important to experience the clinician listening to their concerns from an open and genuinely curious stance, including their hopes and fears for their son's future. The aim of this process and the stance of the therapist is to open the epistemic trust channel, to help parents feel like an important source of information and active collaborators in the therapeutic process. The emergence of epistemic trust opens the possibility of new social learning and generalization outside the consulting room during and after treatment. We reinforced the attempts by Michael's parents to understand their child from a humble and genuinely curious stance. They talked about Michael as a person with his own vulnerabilities and strengths, his problems and needs. Their efforts to give Michael all the chances to grow and develop were clear. When assessment can be carried out within a constructive working alliance, it fosters parental mentalizing abilities and helps the family to engage in a therapeutic process (Cregeen et al., 2017). Michael's parents shared later their experience of having left the initial consultation feeling hopeful that this was a place where they expected to find support to understand their complex 7-year-old foster son. In order to facilitate the parents' reflective functioning capacities in this type of work, the therapist attempts to hold the balance between information gathering, reflection on internal experience and creating epistemic trust with all involved throughout the assessment and treatment process (Cregeen et al., 2017).

Assessing parents' mentalizing capacity and the points of breakdown

Even if problems have already existed for a while and development has not run smoothly so far, parents often consult a therapist in response to a recent precipitating event. Request for professional help often indicates that the parent's resources are overwhelmed (Vliegen et al., 2023) and that their mentalizing skills are close to getting lost.

During the first consultation meeting, we therefore tried to learn more about what had brought Michael's foster parents to seek help. They spoke of the patience required with a child that needed intense help with every new developmental task. Until recently, the most difficult part was Michael's unpredictability in what he needed and expected from them, his need for control, and the many conflicts he generated in relationships. The moment they decided they needed help was when he started to throw punches towards his younger brother. Facing worries about being able to protect the children from Michael's aggression and dysregulation felt more difficult than being challenged by Michael's difficult behaviour. This seemed to be the point at which Michael's parents rather stable and strong reflective capabilities were lost, and a need for a quick fix emerged, with them defaulting to more punitive, behavioural ways of responding to his difficulties. Their capacity to think of the child's states of mind as well as their own became impaired, they became parents in "survival mode".

Individual child assessment: when and why?

Given Michael's presentation and history of early adverse relational experiences, the therapist suggested the idea of conducting a child assessment in order to gather information on Michael's developmental mentalizing profile, temperament and emerging personality. They explained to his parents, who had been introduced to the idea of mentalizing, that they wanted to understand Michael's strengths and difficulties as well as getting to know him better. Parents agreed, and three individual child assessment sessions were set with the aim of exploring Michael's social and emotional functioning. Particular attention was paid to Michael's preferred ways of communicating and relating, his strengths and vulnerabilities from a developmental perspective, his readiness and suitability for individual therapeutic work, and the possible ports of entry for therapeutic intervention. In some circumstances, children who have experienced developmental trauma might function in a hypervigilant way, which can create obstacles to conducting individual assessment sessions. In these cases, a family and dyadic focus in assessment might prove more protective towards the child's relational style and lessen the potential fear and sense of threat that the experience of assessment might bring.

His biological parents were teenagers when they conceived Michael, and both had substance abuse histories. Although his mother grew up in a stable and warm foster family, his father had been in and out of foster care throughout his childhood.

Putting the pieces together: from first observations and stories to an assessment of strengths and difficulties

A developmental assessment draws on as wide a range of data as possible (Midgley, 2011), and requires a setting that maximises the amount of information that can be observed (Greenspan & Thorndike Greenspan, 2003). It is important to gather information from key people and settings in the child's life, such as their schoolteachers. Some additional information can come from more formal assessment of e.g. the child's cognitive assessment or from the teacher or a classroom observation. In this case, a series of assessment tools were chosen based on each parent's reports and Michael's overall presentation. A mixture of methods – both structured and less structured – invites the child to symbolise through drawing, playing or talking, and to express themselves about a wide range of themes. This process aimed to help bring together the puzzle of Michael drawing on ideas from psychodynamic diagnostic profiling (Malberg & Rosenberg, 2017, p. 467).

During the first individual child assessment session the therapist used some of the techniques drawn from the time-limited model of MBT with children (Midgley et al., 2017) and asked Michael to draw a house, a tree and a person, and four affect drawings. During the second session, Michael drew his family members as animals, the therapist invited him to tell her why he chose each animal. He also created stories with the help of a narrative story stem task, but his stories were somewhat disorganized and often ended in catastrophe. During the third assessment session, the therapist tried to work together on his genogram and lifeline and engaged in a free play observation; although Michael seemed somewhat anxious, he engaged during the task. Additionally, the therapist took notes about waiting room observations (for further description of these methods, see also Vliegen, et al., 2023, pp. 109–110).

During these activities the therapist attempted to access the child's representation of self and other, as well as to develop a profile of the child which would guide the therapeutic intervention. Additionally, the assessment phase is meant to support the child in a first understanding of the connection between their behaviour – often experienced by those around them as weird, crazy or bad – and what is going on in their mind and body. We aim to foster the child's engagement in the therapeutic process by getting them involved from the very beginning in a playful and flexible assessment framework.

In the context of developmental trauma, relational experiences impact the child's developmental functioning in several domains, and these domains form the background and framework to understand what the child expresses during the assessment. Core topics in the developmental profile that direct our focus can be summarised in Table 2.1.

The following sections provide a detailed picture of Michael's developmental and relational profile.

Attention control, executive functioning, and cognitive capacities

There were initial concerns regarding Michael's capacities to remain focused in the classroom. His parents also reported Michael's high needs to move, jump, ride his bike … in other words to engage intensively in gross motor activities as

Table 2.1 Core topics in the developmental profile of the child.

Developmental domain	Core topics to gather information on
Cognitive capacities, attention control and executive functioning	• Capacity for stress regulation, attention and focus • Intellectual capabilities as assessed in intelligence test or other structured cognitive task • Academic progress and difficulties as observed at home and in school
Affective development and regulation strategies	• Overall mood and emotional tone • Acknowledgement and expression of affects • Central affects • Affect regulation strategies
Representational capacities	• Capacity to be playful, to express themes and to symbolise • Content of play and symbolisation • Capacity to mentalize
Attachment development and relational capacities	• Basic sense of safety • Representations of caregiving relationships • Representations of self-in-relation-to-others • Relationship qualities in relation to significant others • Relational capabilities in relation to the therapist

attempts to engage in bodily regulation, to regain control over what is happening inside his body, perhaps as a way to connect with others from an embodied mentalizing stance. These worries made the therapist consider the first domain of attention in children with complex trauma, that of being able to focus and to learn, of being able to calm down and to regulate arousal and stress. In the classroom, Michael often seemed to "get lost". He sometimes stared for a long time, and the teacher had to "pull him back". The teacher reported concentration problems and general learning difficulties, but she also described him making small steps forward. Doing homework was a big issue. Nevertheless, the teacher called him "a worker and a go-getter". Upon hearing this the therapist thought about his capacity to mentalize at the most basic level, potential triggers to break downs in mentalizing. She was curious about the "getting lost" and considered the possibility of disassociation.

When asked to draw a house or a tree, Michael started immediately. He worked in a focused way and only looked up after the drawing was ready. In other tasks, he required much more effort to start, probably due to the more emotional content. When asked to draw what made him anxious, he put his head between his hands, took his pencil, looked around, put the pencil down again before taking it back and turning it around. He looked away and hesitated … until the therapist proposed: "Maybe you can write down what you are thinking about?"

In conclusion, Michael could be seen as a child whose capacity to focus and to be organized could rapidly change between moments of fleeting attention and moments of being able to focus on a task or an activity. His capacity to focus and learn seemed rather vulnerable and was easily destabilized by internal (for example connecting with affects such as anxiety and thinking about his personal history) and external (being in a new situation at the beginning of the free play situation) circumstances. His longing to learn and his high motivation to focus and to be more organized seemed to go hand in hand with a good capacity to make use of the presence of a caregiving adult – as could be seen during the assessment sessions in his responses to the therapist. This suggested the need in therapy to focus on strengthening his capacity to use his inner resources.

Affective development and affect regulation strategies

His toddler like behaviour, not being able to tolerate a no or a limit, and the difficulty at bedtimes raises questions about difficulties in regulating affect and emotions. Michael struggled when asked to draw about what made him feel scared. It took him a while, before he could write a sentence and read it aloud: "That I will have to go to another school". When asked about the how and why of that idea, he could not expand in drawing or words. He could merely nod and shake his head when the therapist posed yes/no questions.

During the assessment sessions, Michael's difficulties in affect regulation, and the need for non-verbal co-regulation became evident.

At first sight, anger seemed an easier affect to think about than other kinds of feelings. Michael started drawing, remained focused and only looked up again when the drawing was finished, saying "when homework fails again" (referring to the difficulties he had with completing his homework). Invited to tell something more about that experience, Michael responded "I get very angry, then I sometimes throw things on the floor, my pencil or something …" He made eye contact with the therapist for a short moment. Asked what others do in such a difficult moment, he said "they get angry because I don't want to work anymore". When asked whether homework sometimes works out, he answered, "Once I had homework drawing a caterpillar" (colouring parts of a caterpillar as a way to practice multiplication tables). Michael became more vital, as he added spontaneously: "That was really nice homework, I wanted to do that right away". Here, Michael showed some understanding of the impact of mental states on behaviour. This could be considered as a strength in that he actively understood how doing homework was easier when it was facilitated by something he liked to do: practicing multiplication tables by colouring.

Asked to draw something about his sadness, he replied: "When I can't go to my real mom". Asked to tell a little more about it, he replied: "I go to my mom every two weeks". It required a lot of supportive questions accompanied by explicit ostensive cues (smile, tone of voice) to support Michael to think and talk about this. Like putting together little pieces of a puzzle, Michael slowly shared some information through his behaviour and by the feelings he expressed. This process helped the therapist to understand Michael's struggle as he shared how he often cried when he didn't go to see his biological mother, how he played or drew when he was there, that he liked to draw dogs and that his foster mother gave him a sketchbook that stayed in his biological mother's house … When the therapist asked, "Can you tell what is in your head or what you feel inside about that?", Michael only shook his head.

When asked what made him most happy, Michael replied "sports" and immediately started drawing: "Then I'm very happy". He drew quicky and vividly, engaging easily in the activity of drawing and talking about a football match: "This is a football pitch, and I played against the Goal Getters, but we won. At that moment they weren't very good, now they are better!" Here, Michael's capacity to find vitality struck the therapist, while it showed his ability to make use of the secure relationship she steadily offered during these sessions. Michael's capacity to regulate his emotions through physical activity and with the support of a containing and mentalizing adult highlighted the importance of psychoeducation for the adults supporting Michael regarding affect regulation strategies when presented with insecure attachment and difficulties with attention regulation.

Representational and mentalizing capacities, and a pre-mentalizing profile

Michael's strengths and vulnerabilities in the domain of representational skills seemed to be inhibited by the impact of early toxic stress caused by early adverse relational experiences, as can be seen in the rather poor and immature quality of his drawings when compared to those of the average child his age. While drawing a house, a tree and a person, he could say some sentences that refer to a need (the house "is a bit empty, it needs paint"; the tree "really needs water") or to an experience (the tree "was almost blown down once because of too much wind. If the tree gets sick, it will die and they will have to cut it down'; the person "wants to give his mum a hug, his daddy is dead"). Such responses tend to be characteristic of children in which a "psychic equivalence" mode of functioning is predominant, as the boundary between inside and outside is not well established, impacting the child's creative/ representational capacities (Midgley et al., 2017).

When asked to draw his family as animals, Michael started drawing smoothly and with concentration. He drew every family member as the same animal, saying: "I don't know the name" (referring to the animal). "This is my foster mum; this is my foster dad, and these are Carl and Theo. They have the same antlers as dad, but with less … less dashes. Now, I'm going to draw myself." The session continued:

THERAPIST: You are drawing an animal with an antler, and you said, "I don't know the name"?

MICHAEL: Boys like this, girls like that. Different antlers.

THERAPIST: So you are the animal in the upper left, and next to you, those are your foster brothers?

MICHAEL: Carl and Theo, they look the same. They are the same size, and they wear the same clothes … but if Theo didn't wear glasses, they would be exactly the same. There are five of us, three and two equals five.

THERAPIST: Can you tell me something more about these animals?

MICHAEL: They can fight against their enemies, who want to eat them. And sometimes they do accidently, very accidently … kill an insect. Very accidently [yawns].

An important aspect of the development of mentalization in children concerns the integration of the three pre-mentalizing modes and the capacity to come in and out of them by drawing on the child's inner resources and support from trusted adults. A predominance of pre-mentalizing modes as a way of responding to emotional impact can impair a child's development across multiple domains as it blocks and/ or distorts their understanding of themselves, others and the world in which they live. Furthermore, pre-mentalizing modes can often feed into a child's representations of themselves and others as negative and threatening. Because of this, identifying the predominance of pre-mentalizing mode(s) in children who have been exposed to chronic relational trauma is an important focus of assessment. It can guide the clinician's approach to the child. The "teleological mode" tends to manifest where the child occupies a controlling position or displays a need for immediate solving a negative feeling or a problem. In Michael's case, the "sameness" of the animals in the family drawing brings comfort and can be seen as a concrete and teleological way of describing his family members. This goes hand in hand with a rather poor representational quality in drawing as well as in his creative capacity. The end of the story shows how Michael "knows with certainty" (psychic equivalence, expressing the conviction that reality and mental state are definitely one and the same) that there are others that want to fight these animals and that with antlers they can fight back (teleological stance). It seemed that Michael's epistemic hypervigilance was managed by embracing a knowing stance characterized by lack of curiosity and an abundance of certainty. Often, it seemed, this left Michael feeling quite alone with his feelings of fear and loneliness in stressful situations.

When presented with story stems to complete, Michael engaged rather easily, This could be understood as a good indicator of his capacity to represent his internal world through play and stories. However, a conversation regarding his family history and a lifeline was not possible as he became extremely restless and disorganized. A free play observation began with opening cupboards, looking in them, taking and showing objects to the therapist and asking what they were … plasticine, a marble run (a toy that involves building paths and tunnels for marbles), cars, dressing-up clothes … closing the door again and opening another one. Here he seemed to show curiosity and a capacity to ask for help in a trusting way. Then he started a very basic play sequence, but it was difficult to follow:

Michael goes back to the box with the toy animals and brings it to a dollhouse. He takes out some cats and kittens, a dog and a rabbit and puts them in an animal pen. Then he starts a play with the dollhouse that remains incoherent and disorganized.

There is a lot of noise, people seem to be dancing. He is playing on his own, doesn't seem to be aware of the presence of the therapist. He crawls and moves across the floor, making sounds like, *ksst, psst* … He seems to create a scene, is concentrated on what he is doing, but what happens is completely incomprehensible to the therapist. Some dolls fly across the room. When the therapist asks what is going on in the house, there is no reaction. He then suddenly says: "There is another little dog". Michael puts a dog on the roof of the house.

The therapist says, "The dog seems to do dangerous things, just standing on top of the roof?"

Michael makes the figures come down from the roof with a lot of noise. He looks through the chimney, goes back inside the house, makes the *ksst* and *psst* sounds again, then says to the dolls: "What are you doing here?" The dog falls from the roof, and Michael says, "The owner of the dog didn't know he was there."

In this vignette Michael is all over the place, there is no clear sequence in his story, his disorganized and incoherent narrative gives ample indication of the disorganization in his mind: thoughts and ideas jump around, run away with him ... However, the emotional impact of the story was responded to with a teleological response (with characters showing with actions) evident in the content of the play activating a sense of threat. Parallel to this process, Michael's body seemed to mirror his internal disorganization, his posture was tense and lacking vitality, his facial movements oscillated between flat and tense smiles. When asked about his genogram, for example, he became restless and agitated, and could only stammer out a few incoherent sentences. This indicated to the therapist about his fragility and the need to start slowly, helping him to simply pay attention to what was going on in the room and inside himself, working more at the level of attention control to help promote an environment of relational safety where difficult emotional issues could eventually be represented.

Identity and relational capacities

Michael's mixed expectations in his relationships with adults looked like ambivalent attachment strategies. As described in the introduction, Michael would hardly allow his foster parents to care for him or comfort him in difficult moments, whereas in other instances he could be clingy and demanding, which felt "suffocating" to his foster parents. When reunited with his foster mother in the waiting room, he sought intense physical contact, he snuggled up to her, he leaned against her as if he needed to refuel after having been separated. On the one hand, he didn't ask for help at school, but when people were patient and gave him some time and space to find his way, he became more at ease. This could also be seen in the relationship with his foster care worker and his psychotherapist. At home, however, there were moments he could accept help from his parents, although not when stress or emotions ran too high.

When looking at his representations of parental figures in the narrative story stems, Michael's stories were often about parents who were available in a limited way: When a child told his dad there was a monster in his room, or when a child brought a drawing from school, dad said "we don't have time because we are watching a movie". In another story, when a child burned his hand, mother said "That's what happens if you can't wait. Now you must prepare new food." It seemed that although Michael was able to have some epistemic trust in adult caregivers, he failed to sustain it and quickly fell into states of despair and epistemic hypervigilance, registered implicitly in his body without being put into words.

During the assessment sessions, Michael seemed to connect well with the therapist as a new adult entering his life and was able to make use of her presence to cautiously explore aspects of his inner world. Regarding Michael's identity, his story stem stories seemed to reflect his feeling of being an outsider, someone whose care depended on the availability of an adult with a desire to pay attention to his needs. This feeling seemed to be particularly strong when presented with stories which activated both an explicit and implicit sense of threat. In fact, one could only wonder about the impact of the birth of two biological boys in his foster home on Michael's sense of belonging and his identity as a foster child, caught between his loyalty to his biological mother and his foster parents.

A mentalization-based perspective on assessment and developmental trauma

In this chapter we have taken the reader on the first – assessment – part of the therapeutic journey of Michael, a 7-year-old foster child who had experienced developmental trauma. In the final part of the chapter, we want to reflect more generally on how ideas and insights from a mentalization-based framework can help to inform the assessment phase with a child, their parents and network.

Assessment as a dimensional process and its relationship to categorical diagnosis

Mentalization-based therapy for children (MBT-C), as a transdiagnostic approach, is important in the context of chronic relational trauma where there is a need to consider the multiple variables organizing the child's relational and developmental functioning. Assessment cannot be reduced to a process, separate from treatment, ending with a particular categorical diagnosis. A dimensional approach to assessment should lead to a case formulation as it allows for an ever-changing, yet structured picture, one that we often need to revise as the work continues (Muller & Midgley, 2015; Vliegen et al., 2023). This picture shows aspects of the child's internal and external functioning from different perspectives.

It can be difficult to disentangle whether the symptoms of children who have experienced developmental trauma are a direct result of that trauma, or have to be considered as "comorbid" conditions. As regulating themselves and building constructive relations is often difficult for these children, symptoms such as learning difficulties or rapidly switching attention can be seen as ADHD-like hyperactive behaviour; or their social withdrawal, lack of imagination or dissociative moments may seem to be autism-like relational patterns. This renders the assessment of children in the context of developmental trauma even more challenging. Sometimes complementary diagnostic work can be helpful, and sometimes we need to watch and wait.

In Michael's case, we came to understand that his difficulties with focus and attention were strongly linked with his expectations in relationships and how they impacted his sense of safety. He seemed to become more agitated and "hyperactive" whenever he felt confused or doubtful about the intentions of adults. This is important information both diagnostically but also to further inform the potential "ports of entry" for the therapist with this child.

Focus formulation: co-constructing a case formulation

By organising and phrasing the information gathered during the assessment in a case formulation, we aim to *help parents to understand* their child's difficulties in terms of what is happening in the child's inner world. We also hope to be understanding and empathic about how these problems are challenging their parental skills and resources. A dimensional approach that takes into consideration the quality of internal and external representations of relationships, the child's and the parents' mentalizing profile (i.e. predominance of the pre-mentalizing modes in response to emotional impact) as well as the quality of interaction between the child and care-giving adults is central to the development of a working clinical formulation. A case formulation not only includes a picture of the child's developmental func-tioning and of the parents' mentalizing skills, it is also an attempt to guide treatment planning (Malberg & Rosenberg, 2017, p. 466).

In Michael's case, the case formulation highlighted the impact of early developmental and relational trauma on this child's developing sense of self and safety. This pointed to a need to focus any intervention at the level of attention control and trust building, and to support the development of a richer affective world as well as to help him to play and develop an internal representation of adults who are safe and can be helpful. However, the for-mulation also specified the protective factors such as the consistent care of his foster parents and Michael's strong cognitive functioning and capacity for vitality. Another important aspect to consider in the formulation of this case was the need to work with both foster parents in exploring the impact of having their own biological children might have had on their feelings towards Michael and their overall capacity to manage two very different types of parenting styles. Helping these foster parents to mentalize Michael using a developmental trauma lens would be very beneficial in this case.

Why "a shared understanding" can be a challenging endeavour

In practice, working towards a shared understanding between therapists, parents and the wider professional network around a child is a challenging task for two reasons. First, children who have been exposed to chronic developmental and relational trauma often present the therapist with dis-connected and incongruent personal narratives. Moreover, they have had little experience of a trusting adult thinking about their minds and may require a therapist who can model patience, sensitivity and flexibility in interactions. Furthermore, entrusting oneself to an unknown adult is a huge thing to ask from these children, which requires from the foster parents a fair level of emotional balance to enable them to encourage the child in the venture of entrusting themselves to the therapist; and from the therapist a mentalizing stance and growth-promoting interactions.

Second, parents often seek for help at the end of a long searching process, may be referred for psychotherapy in difficult circumstances, and are often during a crisis or are seeking help at this point because of external (e.g. school) pressure. Parents can have unrealistic expectations about treatment as "fixing" their child's problems or can feel hesitant to put additional pressure on the child. Often, some work needs to be done to translate the parents' and/ or referrer's concerns into more realistic expectations about treatment, and/or to co-construct the therapeutic goals.

In Michael's case it would be understandable that his foster parents would expect that all the love and affection they had provided over the years would result in improvement. Psychoeducation about trauma and development can be of great aid to help parents to remain hopeful when facing all the difficulties that come with parenting a child like Michael. In addition, it is important to share a way of thinking about Michael which includes both risk and protective factors, strengths and vulnerabilities. Helping both child and parents to create a narrative through the use of a focus formulation (Midgley et al., 2017), a story that can provide a new way of understanding Michael's functioning and the goals of therapy, is very important from an MBT-C perspective. The focus formulation is the beginning of a co-constructed treatment plan between therapist, child and parents.

The challenge for the therapist: maintaining the mentalizing stance

Working with children who have endured chronic relational trauma, requires the clinician to assume a mentalizing stance from the very beginning of treatment, focusing on modelling explicit mentalizing in a benign and often nonverbal manner. This may lower epistemic hypervigilance, facilitate the slow development of both emotional and physical safety and set the base for the development of new ways of interacting which promotes connection and safety in relationships. Asking ourselves in what context the child mentalizes best is an important assessment question which will facilitate both clinical formulation and treatment.

The main aim of MBT with children is to provide the child with an experience which promotes the motivation towards connection, safety, and the emergence of (verbal and non-verbal) representation and improved affect regulation. As illustrated in Michael's case, a mentalizing stance from the first sessions helps the whole family regain a positive and hopeful perspective about being able to find better ways of living and interacting. Hope is an important starting point to regain one's mentalizing skills.

In the context of working with children who have experienced chronic developmental trauma, therapists often experience the activation of their own relational past and attachment styles more than in other clinical work. Because of this, it is very important that those of us working in this field are able to ask for help from colleagues and find alternative ways to care for ourselves emotionally and physically. Otherwise, it is easy for clinicians to get engaged in non-mentalizing modes with children, for example becoming emotionally disconnected during play (pretend mode), over-occupied with managing disruptive behaviour (teleological mode) or feeling sure that only we know what is going on for a child (psychic equivalence).

Considering the emotional impact of this work on our own capacity to mentalize, it is important to apply multiple lenses, including one's own self-observation from the outside and from the inside. We must pay attention to the impact of our non-verbal communications as well as sudden emotions that can inhibit our capacity to mentalize children, parents and ourselves. In these moments supervision and team support are essential. It is important that through a mentalizing stance, the therapist learns how to communicate and extend an invitation to think and feel together with parents and children in a sensitive and genuinely curious way (Malberg & Gori, 2024).

Conclusion

The legacy of developmental trauma is often profound, and as the first point of contact with professionals, the way that an assessment is conducted creates an important platform for any therapeutic work to be offered. The process of assessment lays the foundation for a working relationship with the child and parents from which epistemic trust and eventually new social learning can emerge. In addition, a broad, multi-dimensional assessment – making links between behaviour and mental states – seeks to activate the capacity of the various systems surrounding the child to mentalize the whole child. Assessment is the start of an ongoing process, meant to initiate an emerging common vision of the child as well as new awareness and understanding.

As we hope to have illustrated with Michael's case, assessment is a complex process sustained in MBT-C by a series of theoretical and technical principles guiding the observation and interventions of the clinician. A mentalization-based assessment of traumatized children moves away from purely symptom-based diagnosis towards a more dimensional, flexible and accessible map to guide clinical decisions, communications with parents, teachers and other allied professionals. In summary, it is meant to set the foundation for a collaborative intervention in which the aim is to restore, rehabilitate or strengthen a central protective factor, that of mentalization and thus promote development.

Note to the reader

Michael is a composite case in a research project including a manual development of the Psychodynamic Research Team, Clinical Psychology, Faculty Psychology and Educational Sciences of the KU Leuven, Belgium (see also Vliegen, Tang, Midgley, Luyten, & Fonagy, 2023). He is a composite of several children with a similar profile of symptoms and development.

Note

1 Michael is a composite case in a research project including a manual development of the Psychodynamic Research Team, Clinical Psychology, Faculty Psychology and Educational Sciences of the KU Leuven, Belgium (see also Vliegen, Tang, Midgley, Luyten, & Fonagy, 2023). He is a composite of several children with a similar profile of symptoms and development.

References

Cregeen, S., Hughes, C., Midgley, N., Rhode, M., & Rustin, M. (2017). Short-term psychoanalytic psychotherapy for adolescent depression: Framework and process. In J. Catty (ed.), *Short-term psychoanalytic psychotherapy for adolescents with depression: A treatment manual*. Karnac Books.

Greenspan, S. I. & Thorndike Greenspan, N. (2003). *The clinical interview of the child*, 3rd edition. American Psychiatric Press.

Malberg, N. & Gori, I. (2024). Epistemic justice and neurodiversity: Mentalization–based treatment with children in the autistic spectrum from a dimensional perspective. *Journal of Infant, Child, and Adolescent Psychotherapy*, 23 (1), 56–71. doi:10.1080/15289168.2024.2306460.

Malberg, N. & Rosenberg, L. (2017). Profile of mental functioning for children. In V. Lingiardi & N. McWilliams (eds), *Psychodynamic diagnostic manual*, 2nd edition. Guilford Press.

Midgley, N. (2011). Test of time: Anna Freud's *Normality and Pathology in Childhood* (1965). *Clinical Child Psychology and Psychiatry*, 16 (3), 475–482. doi:10.1177/1359104511410849.

Midgley, N., Ensink, K., Lindqvist, K., Malberg, N., & Muller, N. (2017). *Mentalization-based treatment for children: A time-limited approach*. American Psychological Association.

Muller, N. & Midgley, N. (2015). Approaches to assessment in time-limited mentalization-based therapy for children (MBT-C). *Frontiers in Psychology*, 6, 1063. doi:10.3389/fpsyg.2015.01063.

Vliegen, N., Tang, E., Midgley, N., Luyten, P., & Fonagy, P. (2023). *Therapeutic work for children with complex trauma: A three-track psychodynamic approach*. Routledge.

Chapter 3

The assessment of parents and carers of traumatized children

Karin Ensink and Jordan Bate

For children who have experienced early developmental trauma, the capacity of parents and carers to provide safety, and show love, understanding and support, is central to their recovery. Children with histories of trauma may present with challenging reactions that are unexpected and difficult to understand and to respond to. The challenges can be even greater in the context of attachment disruptions, when a child is being cared for by someone new who doesn't know them (i.e. a foster parent or kinship guardian) and may have their own hopes and expectations about fostering a child. Past trauma or adversity in a parent's own life that has not been adequately mentalized may also interfere with that parent's capacity to respond sensitively to the child's distress or anger, as it may reactivate the parent's trauma-related affects. The parents' personalities, their expectations, mental health and attachment styles may also influence their emotional and behavioural reactions and responses to the child.

When these children are referred to therapeutic services for help, the purpose of the assessment is to identify the abilities and challenges for parents in their attachment relationships, to support them in fostering greater security and reflective functioning that will help children recover from trauma. Parents have differing capacities to understand the psychological experiences of children, and to look behind the behaviour of children to think about what it says about trauma-related feelings such as anger or fear. This chapter describes the assessment in two cases – Frankie's foster parents and David's mother – which are fictional composites that are based on families seen in an outpatient clinic in a North American city, using a mentalization-based framework. In both cases, the therapist working with the parents was the individual therapist for the child (in contrast to models where there is a team of two therapists treating the parent and the child).

Assessing the parent's perspective of the child's difficulties

In exploring the presenting problem and the child's developmental history, we observe the parent's mentalizing capacities when talking about their child and encourage them to identify and discover the child's strengths, or what the

DOI: 10.4324/9781032713441-6

parent sees as their "vital spark." As parents begin talking about the struggles with their child, the therapist aims to develop an understanding of the following: (1) the child's difficulties, including when they started, their frequency, and what tends to help or make things worse; and (2) the way the parent understands or misunderstands and responds to the child and the child's difficulties.

Some behaviours become more problematic because they are misinterpreted by parents. For example, the child may be perceived as intentionally defying or attacking them. In the context of fostering a child, the foster parents may be confronted with child behaviours that are difficult to understand, overwhelming and bewildering. The feelings evoked in carers by these behaviours, such as rejection, helplessness, resentment, fear and anger, may make it even harder to understand and imagine what may be happening inside the child and the distress their behaviours may express. Parents may fear that these problems are going to go on forever, or that they are incapable of adequately providing for the child what they need, or that the child is irreparably damaged.

Parents who have unresolved trauma may experience particular challenges dealing with dysregulation and anger in children with developmental trauma. Our research has indicated that parents who have experienced trauma but who were able to mentalize trauma and consider the impact of the trauma on their personality are able to protect their children and establish organized attachment relationship with their children (Berthelot et al., 2015). Parents who have not adequately mentalized past trauma and its impact on their personalities are more likely to have children with disorganized attachments. This suggests that trauma that has not been mentalized, can negatively impact parenting and can contribute to attachment disorganization. Furthermore, we have found, in the context of child sexual abuse, that parental reflective functioning as well as the capacity of parents to establish secure attachment relationships have a protective effect (Ensink et al., 2017a, 2017b). Fear and aggression activated by the child's aggression may make it difficult for parents who have experienced trauma themselves to see the child's distress. The child may in turn feel abandoned and become even more dysregulated. Identifying this dynamic may help both parent and child to mentalize this *interactional pattern* so that it does not turn into vicious cycles of escalation of dysregulation which can interfere with the way parents see the child and understand their difficulties. A parent's own trauma and loss that has not been mentalized can also lead to blind spots where they don't see danger (for example that a partner or friend behaves inappropriately to their child) or are blind to the way they themselves may be perpetuating intergenerational cycles of trauma. While such dynamics may be perceptible to the therapist in the first meeting, the therapist needs to mentalize when and to what extent this will need to be brought to the parent's attention so that they can become more aware and find opportunities to interrupt and change the pattern.

During the assessment process, therapists need to be aware of the level of epistemic trust and vigilance present in the therapeutic relationship and notice when there are breakdowns in trust. We have to remember to put ourselves in the parents' shoes and imagine how challenging the situation is. We may notice that a parent seems to have their guard up and are careful about what they are saying. Parents whose children have experienced attachment trauma may be particularly concerned that they will be blamed or may blame themselves and feel that they have failed their children. Mentalizing the parent and emphatically validating their experience in these moments can help to reopen the channels of communication and encourage them to talk openly. The therapist must also be aware of their own epistemic trust, whether they are open to learning from the parent or if they are becoming judgemental. While these reactions are understandable the therapist needs to notice this experience in themselves so that they can make sense of it and use it clinically.

Understanding the parents' understanding of the child's difficulties

The first case we will use to illustrate the assessment process with parents is Sonia and John, foster parents of an 11-year-old bi-racial (Black and Latina) girl, Frankie, whom they were planning to go on and adopt. Sonia is White and John is bi-racial (White and African-American).

Frankie was referred to treatment by her foster parents and the foster care agency because of concerns about her behaviour in the context of changing homes. The vignettes are presented to provide a picture of how the assessment with the foster carers unfolds. Inserted in brackets throughout are notations about the process, annotating how the concepts outlined in a mentalization-based approach appear in clinical work.

THERAPIST: Why don't you start by telling me a bit about Frankie, and how you came to be parents? [The therapist begins with openness and curiosity, evaluating the current situation and also creating a narrative.]

SONIA: Frankie has been with us for about six months. We took her and Jack, who is five, as a pre-adoptive placement. They were in kinship care with their godmother since they were very young, and they've had a relationship with their mother, but she has not been able to remain sober, so the goal was changed to adoption. That's what led to them coming to us. Their godmother is getting older and has health problems so she did not feel she could adopt them. The first few months were the pretty classic honeymoon phase, but now we are starting to see some behaviours come out and we think it's probably important that she has a therapist.

[The therapist notices that Sonia has given the facts of what has taken place, and as the parents go on to describe Frankie's behaviours, the therapist will attempt to assess not only "what happened" but also "what the parent makes of it," "how they feel," and "how they think their child feels."]

THERAPIST: So, things are moving toward adoption, but you have also been noticing things that you are concerned about. Tell me more.

SONIA: It feels like there are two different Frankies, or maybe even three. I'm trying to think about where to even start. [Suggesting that the parent feels somewhat overwhelmed by the magnitude of the difficulties.] She's always had trouble with bedtime, but now we have to stay with her for hours. We try to do our bedtime routine and then leave but she won't stay in her room. She comes out and pleads with us to stay with her or to be allowed her tablet, she wakes up her brother. We don't know what to do at this point. We know that this is hard for her and want to help her through it. So, we spend hours with her, sitting in her room, which we try to do quietly. But I can't tell if it's helpful or just enabling her. And it's starting to spill over into other things. Like if something isn't exactly how she wants it, she will throw a fit and need us to help her fix it right away. We know that routines are important, and she needs control and has so little control right now, so we try to do things as she wants, but it's just impossible. We don't know what to do at this point. [Sonia tries to consider Frankie's internal experiences, wants, and needs, and wants to respond in a way that is helpful to her. She is open about the difficulties she has with knowing what to do.]

THERAPIST: It sounds like you've been thinking a lot about her needs and feelings amidst these challenges. How are things in other areas of life, like does she have friends? How does she do in school? [The therapist is showing interest and curiosity, validates the mentalizing of Sonia and underscoring that people can be different in different situations.]

JOHN: She is really smart, but in the past, she has thrown chairs and had to be removed from the classroom. That hasn't happened since she's been with us. She has a couple of good friends in school, but I worry about that too as she gets older. If she's in charge it's OK, but I am just thinking about how it seems like more and more she needs to get her way.

THERAPIST: I get it that you are worried that this may become a pattern, rather than some passing phase, and you are questioning your behaviour and worried that it may reinforce this pattern, rather than help her to become more secure and calm. Would that be fair to say?

Through listening to how the parent responds to questions like these, the therapist is thinking about the parent's mentalizing, and whether the parent has a balanced representation of the child, that includes both their difficulties and their strengths. In this case, Sonia can think from Frankie's perspective and imagine what she may be experiencing. Sonia tries to set boundaries but remains flexible and does not become judgemental, she is genuinely concerned about Frankie's development and seems trauma-informed. We get the impression that her mentalizing is solid and there is nothing apparent in the parent's reactions or expectations that is escalating or maintaining Frankie's difficulties. As Sonia notes, Frankie has not had a breakdown at school since she is with them, suggesting that in some ways Frankie is feeling more contained and is responding to the security and care that the foster family is providing. At the same time, the foster parents need help in mentalizing why bedtime may be particularly difficult for Frankie. She may still be hypervigilant, fear abandonment, or find it difficult to be alone with her thoughts and feelings. Understanding this may at least help the parents to not feel personally responsible for the child's behaviour or feeling that they are doing something wrong. While the parents may be able to understand Frankie's behaviour, they will also likely still need space to talk about their internal experiences, including their feelings in the moment, such as their concerns that they are inadvertently encouraging her behaviour. Parents, like Sonia and John, may start with a specific difficulty in how to handle bedtime, but may then reveal deeper concerns about the child's difficulties and evolving personality. The therapist notes this; further questioning may investigate and help the parents think of whether Frankie has other positive interpersonal qualities that go unrecognized when the parents feel at their wits' end.

It is much more difficult when the foster parent has unrealistically high and rigid expectations and sees a child's difficulties as a refusal or defiance with the implication that the child is intentionally doing something that they should be able to control. In such cases, the therapist tries to better understand what the obstacles are to letting go of unrealistic expectations, to help the parent adjust these expectations.

Assessing the parent–child relationship and parenting

We assess the parent–child relationship to identify potential ways in which we can support parents to provide care for children who may present with disorganization and dysregulation. We use three methods: (1) observation of how the parent and child interact in the context of the intake interview; (2) semi-structured interview with the parent, the Parent Development Interview (PDI; Slade & Sleed, 2024); and (3) observation of a structured task, the Squiggle Parent–Child Interaction Task (Ensink et al., 2017b). We utilize these assessments to identify the parent's mental representation of the child, and their capacity to understand the child as a distinct psychological being with a personality. We examine whether the parent can consider the impact they have on their child and the feelings this may evoke in their child, or do they think of the relationship mainly in behavioural terms and right or wrong. We are also concerned when we notice angry preoccupation about a behaviour or a minimization of the child's experience.

During the intake interview. Frankie, her mother, and her father attended the second session together. When the therapist came out to the waiting room, Frankie was snuggled up against her foster mother, Sonia. Sonia held up the phone to the therapist and said, "We are trying to decide which Addams Family movie to watch, the old one or the newer animated one." Frankie's foster father is sitting on the other side of Frankie but is not engaged in this with them.

THERAPIST: Hello Frankie, glad to be meeting you today and seeing you together. Please make yourselves at home. We can all talk together, or as you can see, I have toys and games and some craft things. What do you think? [Therapist is showing genuine interest.]

FRANKIE: Do you have paint pens? I like paint pens.

THERAPIST: Hmm, I don't think I have paint pens, but I think I have markers and crayons.

FRANKIE: [Looks angry and pouts.] Not as good.

THERAPIST: Yeah, I know, I have seen paint pens, they're pretty cool. I'll get the stuff I have out, just in case you decide you want to use it. How about you, Mom and Dad, do you draw? Or what do you like to do? [Offering Frankie the possibility to choose which fosters agency; trying to create we-ness.]

SONIA: I can get into drawing, I'm not as good as Frankie, but.

JOHN: I haven't drawn in a while, but I can if Frankie wants to.

THERAPIST: So, I'll start with some talking and we can draw at the same time. How does that sound? [Drawing helps to reduce the intensity, regulate emotions and provide different channels of communication.]

FRANKIE: OK.

THERAPIST: OK. Well, I guess we should start with, do you know why your parents thought we should meet today? [Asking Frankie about expectations of the session and showing curiosity in what Frankie thinks about coming to therapy; recognizing Frankie by pitching the communication in the room at her developmental level from the start.]

FRANKIE: Yeah, because kids in foster care should have a therapist for their feelings.

THERAPIST: Well yeah, that is one reason kids come to see me, for their feelings. So your parents think you might have some feelings because you are in foster care? [Being explicit about the foster care helps to bring in reality.]

FRANKIE: Yeah. Can I draw? I don't want to talk. I don't like talking about my feelings. Well, it's not that I don't like talking about them in general, but I don't like talking about them to therapists.

THERAPIST: Oh, so it's annoying to talk to pesky therapists, I am not the first therapist you've met with. [The therapist is using humour to talk about herself and validate Frankie's wish to not talk too much.]

FRANKIE: No, I've had a bunch of therapists, and they don't do anything. We just do boring stuff and then they leave.

SONIA: There was one therapist you kind of liked, right? Madeline?

FRANKIE: They all say you can trust them, and they will help, but you can't trust them.

THERAPIST: Ah, you were disappointed and had your trust broken. I understand that would be annoying and hurtful. [Trying to understand the feelings of Frankie and naming possible different feelings helps give meaning to her behaviour.]

SONIA: Well, this is a fresh start.

We notice Frankie's foster parents getting involved while Frankie pouts somewhat angrily. The carers' efforts seem to work to some extent. When Frankie dismisses the therapist, Sonia reminds Frankie of positive experiences she has had. Again, when Frankie says she does not trust therapists, Sonia tries to suggest that she has the chance to make a fresh start. Frankie tries to control the situation by resisting engagement with the therapist but then starts talking and expressing her anger about not being helped. We wonder whether Frankie both longs for security and is angry and bewildered about losing her attachment figures and may want to control her current relationships to avoid loss. We can imagine that it can be challenging for the foster mother, to shift from cuddling with Frankie in the waiting room to dealing with a pouty child who rejects other attempts to engage. We have in mind Sonia's concern that she may be inadvertently encouraging Frankie's controlling side. The therapist wondered about the foster father whose presence at the session suggests that he is there to support his family but might feel excluded or fear intruding. She makes a note to follow up with him about this and wonders whether Frankie may potentially respond differently to him than to a female caregiver. His less emotional style may help him to be less affected by Frankie's tendency to be controlling, and more matter-of-fact about limits in a way that might help contain her anxiety.

Using the squiggle task to help assess parent–child interaction

The squiggle task (Winnicott, 1968; Ensink et al., 2017b) involves the parent and child making a series of six drawings together. First, the child starts a squiggle, which the parent completes; then the parent starts a squiggle and the child completes it; and so on. They number the completed squiggle as they go, and once completed, line up the pictures and take turns telling a story. In terms of mentalizing, the parents' reflective capacities can be observed "in interaction" through their direct communication with their child, their nonverbal communication and responsiveness, as well as in their ability to make meaning of the child's squiggles and construct a story that reflects an understanding of what is meaningful to the child.

The squiggle task provides an opportunity to observe parent–child interaction more directly under the stress of having to structure and direct the child and complete a task together. We observe whether parents provide adequate structure and directions, engage the child's interest, provide encouragement, and refrain from criticism. We are also able to observe whether the parent can mentalize and use their knowledge of the child's experiences and preoccupations to create something meaningful in the process and interpret their squiggle. We consider the parental mentalizing assessed by the task as central to the parenting of children with attachment trauma, where the parent is challenged to understand the child, see their behaviour in terms of what it communicates of their psychological experience, and help the child make meaning and understand their experiences.

The squiggle parent–child interaction task is especially useful in contexts where there are concerns regarding good-enough parenting and the capacity to engage with the child to support their recovery. In these contexts, it may be impossible to obtain the information we need about parenting through direct questioning; some parents may be defensive or may lack the mentalizing capacities to know that they are not responding adequately to the child's physical, emotional, and attachment needs, or that their responses to the child's reactions are inappropriate.

David, a 6-year-old, White American boy, was referred to therapy by child protective services. He currently lives with his mother, Jennifer and his 2-year-old brother in a shelter that is specifically for women and children who have experienced domestic violence. Jennifer and David's father, Paul, had a high degree of conflict in their relationship and both parents had verbally and physically abused each other, but not the children. His parents are both white American. During one of the early parent–child assessment sessions, we introduced David and his mother to the squiggle task.

In David and Jennifer's squiggle, we saw that Jennifer could confidently direct David to engage in the activity. She was playful and creative in making a squiggle to begin with. She took the lead in saying what comes next and David followed her structure. He enjoyed engaging with her in a mutual activity. She was encouraging and reassuring when he was hesitant. She made the effort to understand, "read" into and make something of David's squiggle. She made meaning of his squiggles in a way that showed that she was in touch with his psychological experience and preoccupations. She took up the theme of David's favourite game character, "Mario the survivor", and his capacity to drive through fire and not die, a story which David is intrigued by and has symbolic significance for him, possibly because he identifies with the little guy and has survived the "fire" of his father's violence towards his mother. David expresses delight in this and gets involved, elaborating the story further. The therapist has the impression of a child who feels that his mother "gets" him and a parent who is able to interact with her child in an attuned way.

Clinical use of the Parent Development Interview

In addition to directly observing the parent–child relationship, we seek to understand parents' representations of the relationship. The Parent Development Interview has proved valuable to therapists in assessing parenting in contexts where children have experienced relational trauma or where there are parenting concerns (Slade & Sleed, 2024). A key aspect of the interview is that the parent is asked to pick three adjectives or words to describe the relationship with their child and then to give examples of specific memories that would illustrate why they chose each word. They are also asked to describe their child, in terms of the kind of person they are, and provide examples. The interview goes on to explore the parent's experience of parenting, including what worries they have, what gives them pain or difficulty, and what brings them joy. The assessment covers the parent's ability to recognize the signals of the child when they are distressed and need help and what this communicates about what the child feels and needs. We also ask parents to describe themselves, and what kind of person they are. This allows us to assess the parent's capacity to self-observe or their mentalizing regarding self.

The therapist observes whether the parent has a solid ability to mentalize themselves and their child. Sometimes parents may have generally underdeveloped mentalizing, or the parent may have a higher capacity to mentalize, but certain contexts may impact on their mentalizing capacities. They may find certain experiences easier to talk about. A parent may eagerly talk about the joy they experience but have difficulty articulating times they experience pain, or vice versa. While we prefer to notice and nurture the positive efforts parents make, it is the therapist's responsibility to identify difficulties and failures of parental mentalizing that can negatively impact the child, such as:

- developmentally inappropriate expectations of the child;
- misattributing negative intentions to the child;
- overly negative representations of the child as bad, a failure, for example "just like their father";
- insisting that only behavioural solutions such as physical punishment are effective because the child needs to learn that the parent is in charge;
- detailed descriptions of the child in a way that does not connect with affective experiences; and
- disengagement from the parental role and ignoring the child's distress or bids for interaction.

Assessment of trauma with parents

During the assessment phase, we assess the parent's history of trauma and adverse childhood experiences and ask parents about the trauma their children have experienced. A semi-structured interview covering adverse childhood experiences (ACEs) integrated as part of the standard procedure can be helpful. Questions may include:

- What impact have these experiences had on your personality?
- What would you say you have gained or learned from having the kind of upbringing you had if anything?
- Why do you think your parents behaved as they did during your childhood?
- How do you think your experience as a child being parented the way you were affects your parenting now?

When parents have been in abusive relationships, we start with exploring the impact of these proximal experiences, before moving to their earlier experiences of abuse and neglect. Once the parent has shared their own history of abusive childhood experiences, it may be easier for them to answer the questions for their child and understand that these questions are being asked to keep their child safe, not to be critical of their parenting.

In wrapping up an assessment of trauma it is helpful to come back to the question of who in their own life has had a positive influence on them and help them identify potential "angels" in their histories (Lieberman et al., 2005).

In the case of Jennifer, the mother of David, in the initial intake meeting she had mentioned having her own experiences of maltreatment. When meeting with her, as part of the assessment, the therapist took time to reflect with her on what happened in her own life, offering her the experience of having someone who can hear her story and understand where she is coming from, before supporting her in reflecting on her child.

THERAPIST: We have talked about your relationship with Paul, the chaos and fear, as you described it, and the abuse you experienced, which I would consider a traumatic experience, would you? [Being curious about the emotional impact of the experiences on Jennifer.]

JENNIFER: Oh yes, I mean, I've been through a lot of trauma. I have PTSD from it. I don't even know where to start. I've been raped, I was sexually abused as a child. My mom was in abusive relationships, I saw her get abused. I was abused by her boyfriends.

THERAPIST: These experiences leave a mark on us. [The therapist combines empathic validation and gives a little bit of psychoeducation about intergenerational trauma.]

JENNIFER: Oh yeah, it left marks alright. I mean, I never had any template for a healthy relationship with a man. Except maybe my grandparents.

THERAPIST: And now you are raising two boys. [The focus is on parenthood.]

JENNIFER: Yeah, that's why I don't want them to focus on what they've seen from their dad. I want them to be different.

THERAPIST: I want to come back to that, what you want for them. But going back to you for a second, you had a difficult childhood. How did those experiences impact you as a child, but also as an adult, your personality? [The therapist validates and parks the statement of Jennifer about what she wants for her children, because she wants to focus on the mother first. Asking about the impact is a reflective question and the therapist then listens to what is said and how it is told.]

JENNIFER: I was scared. But I also always saw myself as older than I was. I knew how to take care of myself. It got me in trouble when I was younger when I lived with my grandmother, and she made me go to therapy because I wasn't following her rules. I was going out, staying out with friends, doing stuff I shouldn't have been doing.

THERAPIST: It sounds like you had to grow up fast, taking care of yourself in a way that kids shouldn't have to. That can be tough. You mentioned that your behaviour led your grandmother to send you to therapy. How did you feel about that? [Empathic validation, curiosity and asking for clarification]

JENNIFER: I hated it. I was angry, and I didn't want to be there. I felt like no one understood what I was going through, and I didn't want to open up.

THERAPIST: When you're trying to protect yourself, it's hard to let your guard down, especially with someone you don't know. [Combination of empathic validation and psychoeducation.]

JENNIFER: Yeah, exactly. I didn't trust anyone back then, and honestly, I still struggle with letting people in.

THERAPIST: I hope you're feeling OK with me, I understand you don't know me and have much reason not to trust me. I appreciate how much you are sharing. [Empathic validation in combination and mentalizing the relationship]

JENNIFER: I know. I'm trying. I just don't want to mess them up, you know? I want them to have a better life than I did.

THERAPIST: And when you were young, who did you turn to when you were hurt? [The therapist tries to keep the focus of the conversation on Jennifer herself].

JENNIFER: I mean, no one. There just wasn't anyone.

THERAPIST: How about now? [Switching between past and present offers the opportunity to notice differences, offer hope for change, build coherent narratives and highlight developmental progress.]

JENNIFER: Now? I didn't think I would say this, but I guess my mom. She's chilled out a lot, and she helped me see that I needed to get my kids out of that situation.

The therapist went through a checklist of adverse childhood events with Jennifer, who stated that she had been physically, emotionally, and sexually abused and neglected as a child. After going through these questions and giving Jennifer the space to elaborate where she wanted to, the therapist shifted gears to ask the same set of questions for David.

THERAPIST: So now I'd like to go through this same set of questions, but this time will ask you what David has experienced. Since David was born, did a parent or other adult in the household often or very often swear at him, insult him, put him down, or humiliate him? [Knowing more details about the violence a child has experienced can be helpful in addressing the trauma triggers in the child therapy.]

JENNIFER: I mean he's heard things, but no, it's never been directed at him.

THERAPIST: What about acting in a way that made him afraid that he might be physically hurt?

JENNIFER: I mean, depends on what you consider made him afraid…. if he's really pushing it, I'll remind him to stop, or he'll get popped.

THERAPIST: And for you, what is popped? [It can be a challenge to be genuinely curious as the conversation moves to chastisement and affect rises.]

JENNIFER: Like a smack on the butt, or a smack on the hand if it's something he's touching.

THERAPIST: How often has a parent or adult in the home pushed, grabbed, slapped, or thrown something at him?

JENNIFER: I mean, not often. Maybe a few times I grabbed him or slapped him. But not thrown things or pushed him.

THERAPIST: Ever hard enough that he had marks or was injured? [Talking about violence is difficult and parents tend to minimize the impact of the events because it is so painful.]

JENNIFER: Well, there was one time that I went to grab him, and he pulled away from me and fell back against the table. And he did bump his head then and got a big egg on the back of it.

THERAPIST: Did you go to the hospital or the paediatrician?

JENNIFER: No, it wasn't that bad. But definitely, I was scared at first and didn't know what would have happened if I had needed to bring him. I felt so bad.

THERAPIST: When was this?

JENNIFER: This was when we were still living with his father, like maybe a year or so ago. I was not in my clear mind.

THERAPIST: Got it. And I do want to just say at this point, I do want you to be able to talk openly with me about how you're doing and how things are going so that I can help you have the support you need so that you don't get to that point and if you are getting to that point, we help you. So both you and the kids are safe. [The therapist tries to create a context in which possible dangerous feelings or situations can be discussed openly and without condemnation. This is precisely with the intention that it can remain safe for everyone.]

JENNIFER: Yeah, I mean, I will die if anything ever happens to my kids. They're everything to me.

THERAPIST: [The therapist nods in acknowledgment] In terms of sexual abuse, to your knowledge, have an adult or someone at least five years older ever touched David or had him touch their body in a sexual way? [Naming and looking for possible adverse child experiences can open up the contact because the meta-message is "You can be honest with me. I will not judge you. I try to help."]

JENNIFER: No, definitely not. No to all of these. That's one thing my kids will never experience, I will make sure of it. Because I know it happens to boys too.

THERAPIST: Has David lived with a parent or adult who is a problem drinker or alcoholic or uses street drugs?

JENNIFER: I mean, I drink sometimes with friends. Not really anymore, because the shelter I'm in now is far away from my friends, and I'm trying to keep my distance from their father. And their father smokes weed. I do too, but not ever when they're awake or anything.

THERAPIST: Have you or David's dad, or anyone caring for him, ever been too drunk or high to take care of him?

JENNIFER: I mean, his dad probably, but never when he was alone with him. I was always around.

THERAPIST: Has David ever not had enough to eat, had to wear dirty clothes, or had no one to protect him?

JENNIFER: No, not at all. He's always had enough. I might not, but I make sure he and his brother do.

THERAPIST: These next few questions I sort of know. You and his dad are separated, and there has been physical violence between the two of you. Have either of you ever repeatedly hit the other for at least a few minutes?

JENNIFER: Yeah, the last time, his father hit me hard a few times. I don't know if it was for a few minutes, but it was repeated.

THERAPIST: What about threatening you, or did you ever threaten him, with a gun or a knife?

JENNIFER: His father would threaten but, not with a gun or a knife.

THERAPIST: Where was David when this happened? Did David see or hear this, or try and intervene? [The therapist is not a judge who has to decide on right and wrong, but has a duty of care which includes assessing any current risk to the child.]

JENNIFER: Well, I always told the children to go to their bedroom and close the door. They may have heard but were too scared to come out.

THERAPIST: Would you say that David has lived with a parent or other adult who is depressed or mentally ill?

JENNIFER: I guess me, yeah, I mean I have PTSD. His father I think probably has something. I am pretty sure when he was younger, he was diagnosed with bipolar or something with like anger.

THERAPIST: How often do you imagine that David feels loved, important, or special?

JENNIFER: I hope always!

THERAPIST: Yes! How about that his family looks out for each other, feels close to each other, and supports each other? [Recognizing the positive alongside the negative experiences David has had and the strength of love in the face of adversity]

JENNIFER: Like me and his brother, yeah, and I guess my mom and my family. I think he knows that they're there for him.

When reflecting back on what she had heard from Jennifer, the therapist noted that the risk to her children was low, especially with continued support, but that it could increase if she were to resume contact with Paul and was again subjected to abuse. Jennifer was open about using physical punishment and the matter-of-fact way she talked about it, suggested that she considered it a normal way to discipline children. She admitted sometimes grabbing and slapping David, once resulting in injury when he pulled back and fell. This incident illustrates how easily physical punishment can escalate out of control. Jennifer's concern about this incident suggests that we may be able to help her find other ways of responding that are less likely to lead to escalation of distress and mother–child difficulties, especially as David may start to retaliate. Continuing to work with Jennifer and David, keeping an eye on David, and helping Jennifer talk about her challenges as they arise may seem like a good way forward.

Using the assessment to inform on-going work with parents and carers

The assessment meetings with parents and carers is not only seen as a way of obtaining information about the referred child. Instead, it is an opportunity to develop a "mentalizing profile" of the wider family, and to develop a case formulation, which ties together the reason for consultation with the most salient aspects that have emerged during the assessment. This can help inform the direction of the work with the parents or carers. Usually, the case formulation will not come as a surprise as the therapist takes the parents and child with them during the assessment process, continually sharing and checking their understanding and asking for feedback. In the formulation, the therapist identifies the key difficulties and interactional patterns that the family struggles with and shares goals and objectives in a language that is accessible to the parents and the child. The case formulation keeps in mind the mentalizing capacity of the parents, their capacity to provide parenting that can foster a sense of safety and secure attachment relationships, as well as major obstacles and challenges to this such as unresolved trauma, under developed mentalizing, parental mental illness and previous developmental trauma experienced by the child. The therapist may refer to attachment patterns that may help them think about and understand confusing interpersonal patterns. When sharing a case formulation, the therapist invites the family to correct, change, and contribute to it and makes it clear that they will update the formulation as the therapy progresses and they develop a better understanding.

In the case of Frankie and her foster parents, Sonia and John welcomed Frankie into their home with the hope of one day adopting her and becoming a family. This meant a big adaptation for them and an even more challenging one for Frankie, who had often been let down in her life. While there are many good moments, two main areas of difficulty emerged. Bedtime was a struggle; Frankie struggled at night to shut down, feel safe, and make the transition to sleep, and this was exhausting for her parents and woke up her brother. Furthermore, Sonia was concerned about a pattern of angry, controlling behaviour with her and other relationships and did not want to encourage this inadvertently.

Sonia was loving and emotion-focused, while John had grown up in a more emotionally detached family and had a more straightforward and structured approach to parenting. Sonia shared that she was adopted and always felt a little insecure, trying to please her mother, and not expressing her needs. Furthermore, anger was seldom expressed in her family. She became anxious and fearful when Frankie became angry and controlling and blamed herself for not finding a way of pleasing Frankie. Sonia realized that she was repeating a pattern from the past. The therapist encouraged Sonia to take a step back and helped her consider that even if she did everything possible, she may not be able to please or change Frankie, and this was not her fault. Through taking part in the assessment, the parents came to realize that Sonia's anxious attempts to please Frankie were confusing to Frankie and seemed to contribute to her insecurity as if she was worried that her anger could damage her foster mother. The foster parents realized that they were treating Frankie like a much younger child, and the therapist pointed out that this made Frankie regress.

The therapist empathically validated Sonia's difficulties with responding to anger – it is often the most confusing and difficult emotion for parents to deal with, especially when combined with what they experience as controlling behaviour. She encouraged Sonia to start by simply reminding Frankie when Sonia had to do something and balance her own responsibilities and Frankie's needs, much more typical of parenting a 10–12-year-old. For example, "Remember, I have to get what is on the grocery list and be back to make supper, we don't have time to pop into other shops – will you go find the strawberries for dessert?" Initially, John was unsure of how to get involved, until he discovered that Frankie enjoyed going out with him and her brother to watch sports, swim, or bicycle. Doing this seemed to establish a simpler way of relating for Frankie – for example, John was clear that they did not have money to spend on additional snacks.

As the work continued, both Frankie's and Sonia's moods lightened. The family also slowly found solutions that made bedtime less stressful. Although it was not ideal, Frankie fell asleep on the couch, close to where John worked on his computer in the evenings. This helped her to feel less panicky and learn that it was safe to shut down, let go, and fall asleep in her new house. Eventually, she decided that her bed was more comfortable. Looking back, the therapist reflected that both Sonia and John had good mentalizing capacities and complemented each other as parents, but needed help in navigating the challenges of welcoming a child recovering from painful previous attachment disruptions and help her settle into the family.

In the case of David and his mother, the therapy began with an emphasis on building a safe and supportive environment for both Jennifer and David to recover their sense of security and support them through the challenges of building a new life. The therapist observed that Jennifer had some symptoms of PTSD from recent and past trauma. She feared that her ex-husband would insist on seeing the children or demand shared custody. The work with Jennifer aimed to help her mentalize past trauma and the way this contributed to her fear and sense that she would inevitably become a victim again. The therapist helped her assess her anger about past abuse in the service of protecting herself and her children.

Jennifer also strengthened her ability to mentalize both her own and David's emotions. She realized that she had a traumatic reaction when David became angry and that then she became frozen and fearful and forgot that he was a child. In these moments she was more vulnerable to lashing out and hitting David, as if she was defending herself. Understanding this dynamic of where David's anger triggered her fear and subsequent hitting helped her explore new ways of limit setting that did not involve physical punishment. Over time, Jennifer shared her experiences of trauma and began to explore the deep-seated effects of these experiences on her sense of trust and self-worth, her choice of partners, and her parenting style. Jennifer was surprised that David listened when she set limits verbally and commented that their relationship improved as did his emotional regulation. Rather than see herself as a victim, Jennifer began to recognize her own resilience and strength. She reconnected with more positive aspects of her childhood such as how much her grandmother loved her and helped her. After looking back, she realized that despite the scars that trauma left she was much stronger than she thought and that as an adult she could use her anger to fight back and protect herself and her children in the way she could not as a child. She seemed ready to start planning for herself and the boys.

References

Berthelot, N., Ensink, K., Bernazzani, O., Normandin, L., Luyten, P., & Fonagy, P. (2015). Intergenerational transmission of attachment in abused and neglected mothers: the role of trauma-specific reflective functioning. *Journal of Infant Ment Health* 36 (2), 200–212. doi:10.1002/imhj.21499.

Ensink, K., Bégin, M., Normandin, L., & Fonagy, P. (2017a). Parental reflective functioning as a moderator of child internalizing difficulties in the context of child sexual abuse. *Psychiatry Research*, 257, 361–366. doi:10.1016/j.psychres.2017.07.051.

Ensink, K., Leroux, A., Normandin, L., Biberdzic, M., & Fonagy, P. (2017b). Assessing reflective parenting in interaction with school-aged children. *Journal of Personality Assessment*, 99 (6), 585–595. doi:10.1080/00223891.2016.1270289.

Lieberman, A. F., Padrón, E., Van Horn, P., Harris, & W. W. (2005). Angels in the nursery: The intergenerational transmission of benevolent parental influences. *Journal of Infant Ment Health*, 26 (6), 504–520. doi:10.1002/imhj.20071.

Slade, A. & Sleed, M. (2024). Parental reflective functioning on the Parent Development Interview: A narrative review of measurement, association, and future directions. *Journal of Infant Ment Health* 45 (4), 464–480. doi:10.1002/imhj.22114.

Winnicott, D. W. (1968). Playing: Its theoretical status in the clinical situation. *International Journal of Psycho-Analysis*, 49, 591–599.

Part III

Direct work with the traumatized child

Chapter 4

Working with a toddler

The case of Isidora

Marcia Olhaberry

Introduction

One of the most important tasks of parents is to be aware of their own mental states and those of their children, to sensitively respond to the child's needs and to build secure and reliable bonds. Being born and raised in a family environment where adverse relational experiences prevail can foster confusion, denial, and dissociation, amplifying the sense of threat. In this context, the disorganization of experiences and difficulties in emotion regulation hinder the development of mentalization and increase the risk of presenting with symptoms and mental disorders. These experiences can be understood as traumatic, as the child has been alone when facing difficult emotional situations that have exceeded their capacity to respond.

This chapter presents the application of the time-limited model of MBT in the psychotherapy of a 4-year-old girl with severe regulatory difficulties as a result of developmental trauma. Her parents are separated following a relationship that involved domestic violence, and both have challenging backgrounds, marked by adversity in childhood and the mother's migration from Venezuela to Chile.

Introducing Isidora

Isidora is 4 years old and attends pre-kindergarten at a subsidized private school. Her mother is Venezuelan and arrived in Chile 6 years ago "in search of better opportunities". She has a 9-year-old daughter who lives in Venezuela with her maternal grandmother and did not come to Chile with her mother because "she is more attached to her grandmother than to me" (as stated by the mother). They have weekly phone contact, and due to lack of economic resources, the mother has not been able to travel to visit her. Isidora knows her only through video calls.

Venezuela is going through a complex social, political, and humanitarian crisis that has led 18% of its population to migrate (Human Rights Watch, 2024). Venezuelans constitute the largest migrant community in Chile (32.8%)

DOI: 10.4324/9781032713441-8

(INE, 2023). This situation has generated xenophobia and violent reactions from many Chileans, making it difficult for Venezuelan residents in Chile to access support networks, services, and job opportunities. Migrant families experience grief due to the loss of family ties and significant networks in their country of origin, which can be exacerbated by experiences of discrimination (Pávez-Soto, 2017). In this context, the host country's contextual conditions, including a lack of recognition of cultural identity and social injustices, can lead to mistrust, exclusion, and negative perceptions toward the local population, negatively impacting the adaptation process (Caqueo-Urízar et al., 2019).

Isidora was born in Chile but has not been able to directly meet her maternal grandparents, facing the challenge of integrating two cultures with very different living conditions. Her mother lacks direct family support for parenting, and likely experiences high levels of stress that affect her emotional availability, caregiving, and bond with Isidora. Isidora's father is 12 years older than her mother, and is a teacher. The parents seek consultation at a public healthcare centre in Santiago, Chile.

Parents' concerns

The mother schedules the first appointment and, during a telephone conversation with the therapist, requests not to attend with the father to the initial interview. The father also does not want to attend with the mother, full of suspicion about her motives for seeking therapy. But separately, both agree on the need for psychological help for Isidora. The mother says:

> I am desperate with her, she cries for everything, has tantrums that don't stop, is aggressive with me when I don't do what she asks, and I no longer know how to handle her. When she goes out with her dad, she comes back worse and doesn't tell me anything … I can't take it anymore.

The father's initial concern is:

> Isidora does not respect any boundaries, is capricious, and believes that with tantrums and crying, she will get everything … we already have complaints from the school because she does not work or obey, and she is only 4 years old. We won't find another school that will tolerate her!

From the initial telephone conversations, I see both parents very overwhelmed with raising Isidora, distrustful, and unable to support each other to think about the child and imagine how she feels and what she needs from them. They focus on her behaviour without paying attention to her internal experience, are focused on deficits and difficulties, cannot regulate their own mental states, and are probably unaware of the effect this could have on Isidora. Both make negative attributions about the child and do not seem to be aware of the distress she may be experiencing, especially considering the recent separation, the difficult family history, and the serious conflicts between the parents. I feel invited by both parents to "take sides" for one of them, which makes me imagine the stress and confusion Isidora could feel being in the middle. I feel very pressured and put by the parents in a "judge position" regarding what happened. I am concerned about whether the episodes of violence are current and the risks this could pose to the child. I have doubts about the possibility of initiating a therapy parallel to possible judicial procedures. This leads me to decide to ask supervision for the case. The sessions were recorded and shared with a supervision group.

I start the assessment with four sessions, two with Isidora and one with each parent. In these sessions, I aim to understand the quality of the child's and parents' relationships and their capacity for mentalization, also assessing the connection between reflective functioning failures, lived experiences, and the difficulties Isidora presents. I incorporate several tools to evaluate Isidora's development, identifying areas of strength and areas requiring improvement. For the parents, I use the Parental Development Interview (PDI), recordings of dyadic play sessions with the child (mother–child; father–child), and tools to assess Isidora's socio-emotional and general development (ASQ-SE, ASQ-3). With the child, I use free play, creating a family with animals, and the Completing Attachment Stories for Preschoolers tool. The assessment results reveal significant difficulties in both the child and the parents. For the child, there are traumatic experiences affecting her development and relationships, low self-regulation resources, egocentrism, poor social skills, omnipotence, and a lack of theory of mind. For the parents, there are unresolved childhood traumatic experiences impacting their parenting, low mentalization, low sensitive responsiveness, current interpersonal violence affecting Isidora's upbringing, poor co-parenting, and unresolved attachments. Given the high demand for attention at the health centre and the need for brief, focused interventions, I initially offer 12 sessions for the child and 12 parallel sessions for the parents using the MBT model. Considering the severity of the case, I assume we will need another series of 12 sessions for both child and parents, following review. I also plan to include Isidora in some of the parental sessions to record play interactions, which will later be used in video-feedback sessions with the parents. These session can help to enhance parents observational and reflective skills by providing the opportunity to revisit moments of the relationship in a regulated and supported manner. This is especially used for parents with young children.

Isidora's early years and family history

Isidora is an only child. She lives with her mother and has contact with her father on weekends, sometimes during the day and sometimes staying overnight. They have not been able to establish a stable visitation schedule. They have initiated legal proceedings to order visitation and child support, which are still pending. Due to economic difficulties the father continued to live in the same house for the first 6 months of the separation, but in the child's bedroom. It was common during that period for the parents to alternate between shouting matches and times when they did not speak to each other and used Isidora as a "bridge" to communicate and resolve everyday issues. Many times these fights ended in threats from the mother telling the father "you will never see your daughter again". On one occasion, neighbours called the police upon hearing insults between the adults and the child's crying, which initiated a legal proceeding for domestic violence that ended with instructions for the father to leave the house and a recommendation of therapy for the child. Since that day, the father has been living at his own mother's house, and communication between the parents is mainly through lawyers.

During the first interview with the mother, I explore the child's family history (Lotto et al., 2023). The parents decided to live together immediately and after a few more months they became pregnant with Isidora. The mother mentions a desired pregnancy but with complications from the fifth month that posed medical risks for both her and the child. The birth was highly stressful for both, with Isidora being born at 32 weeks, leading her to stay hospitalized for one month, with visits from her parents restricted to once a day. She was breastfed for 8 months and her further development went well. She started kindergarten at 3 years old because attempts to enrol her at 2 years old failed, with the mother stating that "she cried a lot and couldn't adapt". At the time of consultation, she sleeps with her mother, mentioning that "she wakes up with nightmares at night, the only thing that calms her is sleeping with me … she has always been intense and demanding". She is currently underweight. Mother describes her as "poor at eating, always choosing sweets and junk food". Mother indicates that the separation occurred at the father's decision, and at times, she believes the relationship could be fixed (her eyes fill with tears as she says she still loves him). When asked about the episodes of violence mentioned initially, she says, "all couples have bad moments".

The first assessment session with Isidora

Isidora attends the first session with her mother. Mother insists on accompanying her to the therapy room, saying she will be waiting for her. The girl, annoyed, says, "but I already know that!" She comes with a handbag and lipstick on her lips. I tell her "I see that today you bring a purse and paint lipstick just like your mum", and she tells me, "my mum lent me her lipstick". I introduce myself and ask if she knows why she's here. She says, "I don't know". I mention that I have already met her parents and that they told me they recently separated and don't live together. She turns her back and tries to climb a shelf. I say, "It seems I talked about something that made you feel restless", I approach, tell her it's dangerous to climb the shelf, and not to do it. I offer help and ask her what she wants to take out. She says "I can do it alone". She gets down and goes to the table where there are pencils and paper. She draws circles with a lot of force until the paper breaks. She laughs. I say she "drew with a lot of force, so much that the paper broke". I widen my eyes and exaggerate my surprised expression (using marked mirroring). She looks at me and smiles. She asks for more sheets. I give her two more and she repeats the same thing. I suggest that we could look for a more resistant material than paper to make the same circles or similar figures. She insists that I give her more sheets of paper and says loudly, "my mum buys me all the ones I want". She looks at me and then tears the sheets she drew the circles on. I tell her that I do it differently and that I wonder if that made her angry.

I bring a box of kinetic sand and moulds to play with, inviting her to touch it together. She gets excited, touches it, and says, "these moulds are for me" (choosing the largest ones). I comment "you like the bigger ones", and ask her if she would like me to use any. She says "this one" and gives me the smallest one. I reply that I will only be able to make small moulds in a "complaining tone and expression". She says "because you don't know". While we play with the sand, I ask her if there's anything bothering her, and she says "I don't have any friends at school". She makes sand moulds and then crushes them with her clenched fist. I comment that she hits with a lot of force. She looks at me and then continues hitting. I tell her that I imagine not having friends makes her feel bad. She says "I don't care." I ask her if she wants to tell me about what happens at school with the other children but she doesn't respond. She hits the sand with more force and collapses the remaining moulds. I tell her that maybe I asked a difficult question and that it seems she prefers to play. She looks at me. I ask her what the moulds she makes could be. She says, "poisoned cakes". I ask "for whom?" and she says "for you". I show surprise on my face and ask her "what have I done to deserve poisoned cakes?" (showing surprise and putting my hands on my head). She answers "you behave very badly".

During the session, Isidora struggles to control her impulses and follow any indication or proposal. Her attention span is brief, requiring constant support to stay motivated in a task. She uses the space and materials as if they were her own, without concern for asking or damaging them. These behaviours alternate with a sociable and extroverted attitude, unconcerned about the effects her actions may have on the therapist. In this session, Isidora operates in "teleological mode", expecting the therapist to resolve her boredom, restlessness, and anxiety immediately. She appears omnipotent, demanding, and exigent with the activities, aggressively demanding and competing, trying to resolve internal discomfort with actions.

Given that Isidora's parents primarily focus on behaviour, they have given her few opportunities to learn and express her feelings like when she feels pain, fear, or wants something, having fewer opportunities to learn to think about herself and her behaviours as motivated by mental states. She has been exposed to recurring episodes of violence from a very young age. She struggles to see what she does to trigger reactions in others, only experiencing them as "bad people" for their reactions without understanding how she participates in what happens. The mother tends to act by feeding omnipotence and teleological functioning, while the father responds with severity and disqualifications that increase dysregulation. Children with histories like Isidora's especially need to develop the ability to see themselves from the outside with a favourable view, from a playful context that helps them see their strengths but also their weaknesses.

With my interventions, I aim to establish a bond with Isidora, making her feel comfortable, accepted, and with space to express what is happening to her through different means, in a safe environment. I propose an alternative to scribbling and tearing up the sheets of paper, which seems to be turning into a form of discharge and testing limits, rather than a game that helps her express and identify what is happening internally. I seek a proprioceptive activity to help her relax and allow us to connect. I choose kinetic sand as it allows for creating shapes that can change, is resistant to impacts, and can regulate during moments of distress and stress. Throughout the session, I "notice and name" what I see her doing to achieve joint attention and to help her understand how I see her from the outside and wonder about her. I use marked mirroring to reflect possible internal states of hers, which she projects onto me (not knowing how to make large moulds, deserving poisoned cakes without understanding why).

Through her dysregulation and hostile behaviours, Isidora shows me that putting her experiences into words is very threatening for her, possibly because words connect her directly and intensely with the emotional experience, which disorganizes her (psychic equivalence). The ability to mentalize is especially vulnerable to developmental trauma, and children who grow up in an environment where they cannot trust their parents may seek to adapt by remaining in a state of hypervigilance (Ensink et al., 2014). Experiences of abuse make it difficult to think about oneself and attachment relationships in terms of mental states, which is associated with externalizing symptoms (Ensink et al., 2016), less symbolic play, and difficulties initiating dyadic play (Valentino et al., 2011), as demonstrated by Isidora. In family contexts where abusive interpersonal dynamics occur, low mentalization in parents may also increase the risk of dissociation, interfering with the ability to tolerate difficult emotions and reflect on the consequences of actions (Ensink et al., 2016). This could explain why Isidora closes herself off and loses interest in the motivations and intentions behind my words and proposals. Children who show difficulties in empathy need the opportunity for interactions that allow them to identify other perspectives, challenge them to generate greater awareness of their empathy-deficient responses, and question them.

Reflective functioning in Isidora's mother and father

As part of the assessment, I used the PDI with both the mother and the father. The mother has no idea about the possible influence of her own upbringing in how she is parenting her own child. She fails to recognize that her thoughts, feelings, and experiences during childhood influence her role as a mother with Isidora and therefore the girl's experience of herself and others. She fails to recognize the impact on herself of the sexual abuse she experienced with her stepfather and the shortcomings in her own mother. She dissociates, unable to connect with her own pain, constructing an idea of omnipotent control regarding possible risks to her daughter. She denies the effect of verbal violence and emotional neglect on her daughter operating mostly in psychic equivalence mode.

Isidora's father fails to delve into his childhood experiences or to express his emotions and thoughts in relation to what he lived through with an authoritarian father who physically punished him. He describes parental behaviours and fails to see possible common elements in how he raises Isidora, appearing rigid and rejecting the possibility of considering expressions other than authoritarianism in himself and the effects this could have on Isidora.

When parents show limited capacity to mentalize their child's traumatic experiences, this can have a significant impact on the child's development, personality, and parenting (Berthelot et al., 2015). In the case of these parents, their mentalization capacity is so interfered with that they feel very confident that their ideas correspond exactly to what is happening to Isidora. They may not be aware of their own aggression or the fear this could generate in the child, especially when such fear and anxiety could be related to their own traumas, such as abuse, mistreatment, and abandonment. Their mentalizing is concrete; they only focus on describing the child's behaviours, without showing curiosity about her subjective experience. They fail to imagine the effect of parental separation and aggression on Isidora.

The second assessment session with Isidora: family relationships, attachment and mentalization

In the second assessment session, I decide to use the instrument *Completing Attachment Stories for Preschoolers* (Miljkovitch et al., 2003), since it allows the assessment of family relationships and bonds in a playful way with young children. The instrument involves the therapist telling the first part of a story using dolls, focusing on a particular attachment-related theme, and then asking the child to complete the story. How the child completes each story is very revealing of the child's attachment representations.

When we meet, Isidora goes straight to where the kinetic sand is located, without asking, and says, "We'll make cakes". I tell her that today will be a bit different because I prepared an activity for us to do together at the beginning. She says, "I want to make cakes". I propose a deal to decide what we will play, "for the first half of the time I suggest the activity and for the second half, you tell me what we will play". She agrees but keeps the box with sand nearby. I present the dolls to her and tell her that I will tell her stories that she will have to complete by moving and making the dolls speak. In the first story, she sings "Happy Birthday" enthusiastically with me and adds that the girl ate all the cake and didn't leave any for anyone, she laughs ... and adds that it had poison. In the second story, the father gets very angry and punishes the girl because she spilled the juice, the mother hits the father, and everyone dies (she throws the toys and laughs). In the story of the knee injury, she adds a lot of blood, the girl hits her parents, and everyone dies. The subsequent stories are increasingly shorter and end in accidents and death without options for care or repair. She becomes very restless, with interruptions and complaints about the stories, she wants to take all the materials at once, she struggles to listen to the initial part of each story, she gets up from the chair, and complains that it is too long and it's her turn to "lead", saying, "Your game is boring". I mention that I think these stories were very difficult and I thank her for being able to tell them to me despite that.

Play is a privileged resource in children for dealing with their experiences and creating situations to plan and experience different options and perspectives, making it a highly relevant element for promoting mentalization (Tessier et al., 2016). Conversely, the lack of play skills alerts us to interferences in mental processing and the need for intervention to recover mental processes that may be inhibited (Fonagy et al., 2002). In the stories that Isidora tells, she gets lost in the game, completing the stories rigidly, repeating the endings, and fails to use play to process her own experiences but rather uses it to escape from the reality that each story proposes (committing a fault, injuries, nighttime fear, separations, and reunions). This leads her to dysregulate and quickly need a change of activity. She exhibits elements typical of traumatic play, characterized by repetitiveness, mechanization, and disorganization, with a focus on aggression and harm without possibilities of help or repair (Chazan et al., 2016)

Isidora's experiences from the beginning of her life have generated early developmental trauma that poses a threat to physical and psychological integrity and failures in the social connection system. The stories she tells show extreme aggression and death, lack of parental support, catastrophic fantasies and disorganization that prevent her from creating congruent narratives with adaptive solutions or exits to what the characters face. Her representational models appear constructed from caregivers perceived as rejecting or unavailable, with difficulties in recognizing and validating their needs for protection and care. This could be associated with the construction of a view of "herself" as not very valuable or competent, making it difficult to regulate and interpret and predict the behaviours and mental states of the parents. Since these experiences have occurred with her parents, her ability to reorganize and feel safe and calm again is interfered. The connection with her therapist can be an opportunity to receive care and protection because when she experiences overwhelming emotions she doesn't have much possibility to ask for comfort or repair, as shown in her stories.

Based on my assessment of Isidora's needs, I am aware of the importance of responding with high sensitivity to her communications to help her trust me as a reliable source of information. This also involves building a relationship in which she feels regarded as a child with a "mind", where her subjective experiences are acknowledged, validated, and supported. I demonstrate that I am genuinely concerned about how she "feels inside", understanding the adaptive origins of her hypervigilance and fear of trusting and needing others. My aim is to help her move from the "terrifying certainty" that traumatic relational experiences will be repeated in her new relationships, towards a "secure uncertainty" where she can tolerate not knowing, develop greater trust, openness to social learning and curiosity about mental states in herself and others. From this, I seek to establish a positive therapeutic alliance that aids her in integrating the information gained from her own experiences, relationships, and reality exploration. I hope to help her gradually recognize her emotions, thoughts, and desires in a non-threatening space, facilitating the recognition of the connection between her experiences and the overwhelming and disorganizing internal states that have interfered with her development and relationships.

In the assessment sessions with Isidora, when inviting her to represent each of her family members by an animal, she chooses tigers for herself, her father and her mother. Taking this information into account I propose the focus formulation as: "To find out what is happening with the tigers and discover what they need to feel better." Isidora responds positively to the proposal. More generally, I propose to work with Isidora on improving her ability to regulate emotions, self-observe, and manage difficult aspects of herself (aggression, impulsivity), integrating her lived experiences (domestic violence, parental separation), and enhancing her ability to approach others with a curious and empathetic attitude and learn to make friends. For the parents, the focus is on strengthening parental reflective functioning with an emphasis on relational sequences and co-regulation.

Early phase of time-limited MBT

Towards the end of the sixth session Isidora approaches a basket of relaxation toys. She looks at them, touches them, and chooses a soft, squeezable rubber shark, which she has chosen before. I approach and say, "You like the shark!" She looks at me and says "It has very big teeth to eat with" … She brings it closer to me and says, "It wants to eat you". I respond, "What have I done? [with a surprised look and wide eyes]. I don't want it to eat me, how scary." She smiles and says, "You misbehaved, you wet yourself". I tell her, "Some children have told me they feel embarrassed when they wet themselves and feel sad if they are scolded." She replies, "My mum punishes me when I wet her bed." I tell her, "Perhaps when that happens, Mum looks like a hungry and angry shark and that makes you feel scared and sad". She stays thoughtful.

We are almost at the end of the session and I warn her that "there are a few minutes left before we say goodbye". She gets angry, shouts, and tells me that "it was very little time and that I cheated, that the child before had more time" (she waited with her mother a few minutes in the waiting room). I tell her "It seems like it's hard for you to stop playing today and you'd like to keep playing longer". She looks at me without saying anything. I tell her that "we'll see each other next week". She throws the toys and runs out. She doesn't want to say goodbye.

Through playing with the shark, we could explore Isidora's internal states in a way that is less threatening for her. She places me as the person who will be devoured and that allows me to represent fear. We also explore the reasons for the shark's anger, which allows her to recount an experience of being scolded by her mother and together we find the words to represent how she might have felt. Faced with the limit due to the end of the session, she becomes frustrated and negative feelings are activated in her, leading her to act from a position of "psychic equivalence". She convinces herself of my "bad intentions" and that I gave her less time than other children. Her perception of what is happening becomes distorted by her overwhelming internal states. During this session, I felt stretched and overwhelmed by not having enough time to help Isidora regulate herself before saying goodbye or explore what happened. I am left reflecting on the importance of also considering their experiences in the waiting room and the need for more scaffolding to process these experiences.

Middle phase of psychotherapy with time-limited mentalization-based treatment

By my eighteenth session with Isidora, we had already established a stable structure together. We include an initial greeting, an activity to promote regulation if necessary, a game and a graphic representation of what happened in the session recorded on a calendar. Upon meeting, we greet each other in her chosen manner: Sometimes she waves her hand, other times she says hello, and occasionally she hugs me. I always reciprocate her greeting without favouring one type over another. I acknowledge her chosen greeting ("today you wanted us to greet each other with a hug"), and she looks at me, sometimes serious and sometimes smiling, before we quickly move to the therapy room. Touching children during therapy is a sensitive topic, also in Chile. However, in the context of the waiting room with parents present, greeting or saying goodbye may involve giving a kiss, holding a hand or receiving a hug. Rejecting the hug or touching the hands or the kiss on the cheek could be understood as rejection.

At the beginning of each session, if Isidora "doesn't know what she wants to play" or has "had a difficult week", we sometimes start with a relaxing activity. When she arrives with either very high levels of excitement (restless motor activity, grabbing materials without deciding) or very low levels (lying quietly on the cushions, lost in thought), I suggest using sand, clay, or marbles "to help us feel better". These materials have been effective for her in focusing and regulating emotions. Usually, she starts with kinetic sand, moulding cakes and gradually involving me in the activities, assigning roles (for example, "you eat the cakes"). Then she either chooses what to play or I make a suggestion. This routine provides a secure base, helping her anticipate and better tolerate emotions during our sessions, and manage transitions, separations, and changes from our initial meeting in the waiting room to saying goodbye at the end of the session. These experiences nurture a deeper emotional connection, gradually boosting her confidence, opening her inner world, and structuring her emotional experiences.

After making some cakes and asking me to eat them, she declares, "I know what I want to play now! I need the dollhouse." I mention that it seems like "she feels happy to have an idea for play" and bring the dollhouse closer. She rearranges the furniture, moving it around several times, showing particular interest in the beds and their warmth. I comment that "it looks like she's concerned about everyone being warm and cozy in this house". I ask her "who lives there?", and she stands up to select figures from a shelf at her height: "this is the mum, the dad, and their daughter, a very little baby", placing them in the dining room of the house. I remark, "it seems like it's mealtime for this family", and she tells me "they're very hungry, bring food for everyone and fries for the baby". I find miniature food items and give them to her, and she remarks "they don't like this food". I point out that "they must feel bad not having the food they like". She discusses foods she dislikes, mentioning "Dad makes me eat broccoli and tough meat at his house". I sympathize, saying "I imagine that makes you feel bad when that happens". She doesn't respond, picks up some trees, and places them beside the house, saying "this will be the garden". I observe that "talking about food at Dad's house seems very difficult".

She returns to the house and takes the baby, saying "she felt like vomiting". I ask her if "maybe she doesn't like the food and is afraid to tell Dad", she says "Dad will shout and punish her if she doesn't eat the food". I comment "the baby must be very scared and maybe doesn't know what to do". She looks at me with a sad expression. I suggest that "maybe she felt like this when Dad gave her broccoli and tough meat". She replies, "I cried and asked him to call Mum to pick me up, Dad got angry and they fought". I add "it must have been very sad for her to see her parents fighting". She is silent and takes the baby to the garden. I observe that "when difficult things happen between the parents, the baby seems more peaceful in the garden". She continues decorating and preparing the garden. She seems focused, doesn't assign me a role but seems to enjoy my presence, my descriptions of what she's doing and my questions about the subjective experiences of the characters and the episode with food at Dad's house. Suddenly, she becomes very still, looking at a coat rack. I remark, "I see you're very still and focused on the coat rack", and ask her, "What caught your attention?". She says, "that's Dad's jacket". She stops playing, moves away from the dollhouse and goes to the toy shelf, taking a lace ball with smaller balls inside, trying to open it. I comment "thinking about Dad's jacket made your face change and you couldn't keep playing and preparing the garden". She tells me "Dad didn't come for me and I was waiting", I reply "I think what happened must have made you feel very sad and maybe you thought Dad was angry with you because you didn't eat the food". She doesn't respond, tries to forcefully separate the balls, hits them against the shelf and tells me "this game is bad". I suggest "maybe the fights between the parents make her feel a bit lonely and angry". I approach and offer to help her separate the balls, manage to separate the first two and roll the smaller ball towards her. She catches it, smiles, looks at me, separates the smaller balls and throws it back to me. We repeat the game until we dismantle the lace ball. She asks to play it again several times. I comment "it seems like you were happy that we could play again after remembering something sad that happened with Dad".

As therapy progresses, Isidora increasingly takes ownership of the therapeutic space and shows initiative, developing a trusting relationship that helps her verbalize some personal experiences through play. She is able to identify bodily sensations (like feeling nauseous), and through play and dialogue, connect them with emotional experiences (fear and sadness). Upon seeing a jacket similar to her dad's, she assumes "that's Dad's jacket" and is transported to a painful weekend experience that connects her with conflicts between her parents and the specific moment when her dad didn't visit her. Words seem threatening to process this experience, so through non-verbal communication and establishing rhythms with the ball game, she manages to regulate herself again and connect, possibly feeling contained and accompanied in the painful experience with her father. The final moment of this session shows how extrapolating Isidora's mental states from her body expression (withdrawing from the dollhouse game, taking the ball, being unable to open it and hitting it), adjusting my own movements in tune with her needs (helping to open the balls and creating turns by rolling them), proves particularly valuable in helping her process emotionally disorganizing experiences. This relates to the concept of "embodied mentalization" (Shai & Belsky, 2017), which emphasizes that a child's subjective experience can be expressed in the quality of movement, rhythms, use of space, sensations, and touch.

Despite the progress made by the end of the initial 12 sessions, Isidora begins to exhibit new episodes of dysregulation, but only with her parents, maintaining her progress at school and within the therapeutic space. The relapse is linked to new episodes of verbal violence between the parents, stemming from a legal claim by the mother against the father to increase the child maintenance payments. These episodes and the parental difficulties prompt me to extend the treatment, proposing an additional 12 sessions (Midgley et al., 2017). Simultaneously, both parents were referred for individual therapy with colleagues, with whom I maintained regular contact. The parents' individual therapy contributes to processing the separation and their own histories, improving their parental reflective functioning and sensitivity to Isidora's needs.

Conclusion and final reflections

I worked with Isidora and her parents across a total of 52 sessions: 4 assessment sessions, 24 sessions with Isidora and 24 parallel sessions with the parents. They assisted Isidora in moving from highly frightening mental states from which she could not escape, towards greater security and confidence in understanding herself and others. When she started therapy, Isidora predominantly exhibited a pre-mentalizing state of psychic equivalence as a way of understanding her family environment and the world around her, with difficulties in tolerating uncertainty, being curious, and being open to her own and others' mental states. Her challenges were evident both in the family and social environments. Therapy supported her to develop greater openness to social learning, which also allowed her to develop friendships in the school context.

Initially, due to her history, the initial contact with me was feared, and she exhibited a wary and hypervigilant attitude. This can be understood considering that forming attachments and expressing emotional needs in a new relationship entails the risk of repeating the painful experiences she had with her parents, who were unable to act as a secure base and respond to her emotional needs as she required. Given her age, observing her non-verbal communications, somatic expressions, facial cues, and movements proved particularly relevant during the process as key elements for regulation. The use of my own bodily posture, distance, voice, and movement were crucial elements in restoring synchrony during moments of mentalization lapses.

In her relationship with her parents, tantrums and episodes of intense anger initially decreased significantly after the start of therapy; she began sleeping in her own bed and enjoying her meals. Both her mother and father were able to identify moments when they lost their capacity to mentalize, thereby perpetuating vicious cycles of interaction that heightened Isidora's dysregulation, anger, sadness, and the resulting frustration and suffering for the parents. As a result of the work with the parents, Isidora's mother recognized her own difficulties in organizing and structuring the environment and routines for Isidora, realizing that her own experiences of abandonment and violence hindered her from setting boundaries without feeling like a "bad mother". She succeeded in differentiating her own perspective from Isidora's, integrating elements appropriate to the child's developmental stage and needs.

Additionally, she identified her ambivalence towards the child, acknowledging the anger and sorrow she felt in providing Isidora with the care and protection she had not received from her own parents. Another significant change for the mother was recognizing the need to integrate her Venezuelan heritage into the construction of her daughter's identity. Father was also able to recognize his own severity and harshness in raising Isidora, linking it to his own childhood experiences. He identified the fear his demands sometimes instilled in the child and acknowledged the sadness and emotional distance these episodes created for both of them.

In summary, working with the time-limited model of MBT with a 4-year-old child with developmental trauma involves several key elements. Firstly, recognizing the impact of early trauma on attachment and mentalization is crucial, understanding that actively avoiding mentalization or interrupting the development of this capacity can be a form of protection that help maintain the relationship with primary caregivers. From the child's perspective, mistrust can be an adaptive response stemming from the fear of depending on and needing others, which acts as a shield concealing their vulnerability. These experiences lead children to send messages to keep potentially helpful adults at a distance. In Isidora's case, her strategy for distancing was her "challenging" or "oppositional" behaviours. The child's experience with her parents involved being treated as a child who "makes the father angry" and who is "scary" to the mother, leaving her alone with her terrifying emotional experiences due to domestic violence. This fostered the experience that the relational world is meaningless, unpredictable, or unmanageable, perceived as hostile, humiliating, or persecutory. Restoring trust in others, broken by trauma in both the child and the parents, was a key element in enhancing the positive response to the intervention. In this sense, from the MBT model, therapeutic efforts to reduce threat and fear are central, as well as maintaining a curious and non-blaming therapeutic attitude. When a child is so young and so dependent on the parents as is the case with Isidora, it is necessary to also work with the parents and sometimes work with the parent and child, for example using video-feedback.

Children who have experienced developmental trauma have a tendency to express negative feelings through aggressive acts and positive feelings through overexcitement, with poorly developed emotional language. Due to "psychic equivalence", their play can be very chaotic and destructive, as it is experienced as "too real". They usually have a lower threshold for losing their mentalizing capacity and require more time and support to recover. They need the therapist's support to create a safe space to feel, reflect, understand, and articulate their emotions. From the MBT model, the therapist notices and names what occurs within the interaction, helping to identify feelings (internal experience) and to contain and modulate emotions (visible behaviour). In working on affective regulation, the therapist actively comments on their observations, encourages the child to expand play, sometimes modelling how to play and other times using play to connect words with feelings and sensations. The approach can help the child imagine mental states in themselves and others, based on a secure relationship with the therapist, and take these skills back into their everyday lives.

References

Berthelot, N., Ensink, K., Bernazzani, O., Normandin, L., Luyten, P., & Fonagy, P. (2015). Intergenerational transmission of attachment in abused and neglected mothers: the role of trauma-specific reflective functioning. *Journal of Infant Ment Health* 36 (2), 200–212. doi:10.1002/imhj.21499.

Caqueo-Urízar, A., Flores, J., Irarrázaval, M., Loo, N., Páez, J., & Sepúlveda, G. (2019). Discriminación percibida en escolares migrantes en el Norte de Chile. *Terapia psicológica*, 37 (2), 97–103. doi:10.4067/S0718-48082019000200097.

Chazan, S., Kuchirko, Y., Beebe, B., & Sossin, K.M. (2016). A longitudinal study of traumatic play activity using the Children's Developmental Play Instrument (CDPI). *Journal of Infant, Child, and Adolescent Psychotherapy*, 15 (1), 1–25. doi:10.1080/15289168.2015.1127729.

Ensink, K., Berthelot, N., Bernazzani, O., Normandin, L., &Fonagy, P. (2014). Another step closer to measuring the ghosts in the nursery: Preliminary validation of the Trauma Reflective Functioning Scale. *Frontiers in Psychology*, 5, article 1471. doi:10.3389/fpsyg.2014.01471.

Ensink, K., Bégin, M., Normandin, L., & Fonagy, P. (2016). Maternal and child reflective functioning in the context of child sexual abuse: Pathways to depression and externalising difficulties. *European Journal of Psychotraumatology*, 7, article 30611. doi:10.3402/ejpt.v7.30611.

Fonagy, P., Gergely, G., Jurist, E., & Target, M. (2002). *Affect regulation, mentalization, and the development of the self.* Other Press.

Human Rights Watch. (2024). Venezuela. www.hrw.org/world-report/2024/country-chapters/venezuela.

INE. (2023). *Estimación de personas extranjeras. Residentes habituales en Chile al 31 de diciembre de 2022. Distribución regional y comunal.* Instituto Nacional de Estadísticas.

Lotto, C. R., Altafim, E. R. P., & Linhares, M. B. M. (2023). Maternal history of childhood adversities and later negative parenting: a systematic review. *Trauma, Violence, and Abuse*, 24 (2), 662–683. doi:10.1177/15248380211036076.

Midgley, N., Muller, N., Malberg, N., Lindqvist, K., & Ensink, K. (2017). Mentalization-based treatment for children (MBT-C). In A. Bateman & P. Fonagy (eds), *Handbook of mentalizing in mental health practice*. American Psychiatric Association Publishing.

Miljkovitch, R., Pierrehumbert, B., Karmaniola, A., & Halfon, O. (2003). Les représentations d'attachment du jeune enfant. Développment d' un système de codage pour les histoires à compléter. *Cevenir*, 15 (2), 143–177.

Pávez-Soto, I. (2017). Integracion sociocultural y derechos de las niñas y los niños migrantes en el contexto local. El caso de Recoleta (Región Metropolitana, Chile). *Chungará (Arica)*, 49 (4), 613–622. doi:10.4067/S0717–73562017005000105.

Shai, D., & Belsky, J. (2017). Parental embodied mentalizing: how the nonverbal dance between parents and infants predicts children's socio-emotional functioning. *Attachment and Human Development*, 19 (2), 191–219. doi:10.1080/14616734.2016.1255653.

Tessier, V. P., Normandin, L., Ensink, K., & Fonagy, P. (2016). Fact or fiction? A longitudinal study of play and the development of reflective functioning. *Bulletin of the Menninger Clinic*, 80 (1), 60–79. doi:10.1521/bumc.2016.80.1.60.

Valentino, K., Cicchetti, D., Toth, S. L., & Rogosch, F. A. (2011). Mother–child play and maltreatment: A longitudinal analysis of emerging social behaviour from infancy to toddlerhood. *Developmental Psychology*, 47 (5), 1280–1294. doi:10.1037/a0024459.

Chapter 5

Working with school-age children (I)

The case of Taro

Momoko Nakanishi and Junko Yagi

Introduction

In this chapter, we report a year-long MBT therapy with a 9-year-old boy who had been sexually abused in a long-term neglectful environment. The boy was treated in a Japanese in-patient children's psychiatric hospital unit of a general hospital.[1]

Children with complex trauma often experience epistemic distrust and a negative self-image. Additionally, they live in a constant state of hypervigilance as a defence mechanism for survival. To support children who have suffered developmental trauma and are thought to have had no experience with a healthy attachment relationship, it is essential to approach them from a trauma-informed perspective and with the utmost discretion – like caring for a wounded baby bird. The therapist needs to patiently accompany them through the process of discovering their own emotions and encourage them to trust and connect with themselves and others by supporting their emotional development through repeated embodiment of validation, reflection and empathy.

To develop epistemic trust, it is essential the therapist keeps their promises and is fully present with the children to ensure their psychological safety. In this chapter we have tried to show that the therapist's genuine interest, non-conditional acknowledgement of the child's existence, and the use of carefully considered non-verbal communication can contribute to the child's emotional regulation and sense of being someone. We would also like to emphasize that it is difficult for therapists to keep their mentalizing "online" while working with these children. Thus, therapists need the continued presence of colleagues who can help mutually sustain our mentalizing. Only when the therapist's own mentalizing is online we can feel and express our sincere feelings and thoughts with the child. We also discuss the process of child emotional development and the budding of mentalization in children with developmental trauma; and examine the Japanese cultural context of "empathy", and how this affected our work.

DOI: 10.4324/9781032713441-9

Background information

Taro's mother, who had a history of adverse childhood experiences (ACEs) and sexual abuse, gave birth to Taro as a result of a casual relationship with a man she met on a social networking site. The biological father did not acknowledge Taro's paternity and left the mother shortly after she became pregnant. Due to the mother's neglect caused by her depression and emotional instability, at the age of one Taro was taken into temporary care, then placed in an orphanage, as is quite common in Japan for young children removed from their parents' care. The mother's visits were irregular and she often didn't show up on scheduled visitation days. Taro's mother took him back in when he turned five, but six months later the police had to assume temporary custody after they found Taro wandering around alone at night. Interviews revealed that a man the mother was involved with had physically and sexually abused Taro. After re-admission to a children's home, Taro often threw violent tantrums and suffered from insomnia and enuresis. His mother was also hospitalized for mental health problems and repeated suicide attempts, so her visits were restricted. Taro was eventually transferred to another institution once it was discovered he had been engaging in sexual interactions with children of the same age (touching each other's private parts).

Due to various problems, Taro was admitted to a child psychiatric unit at the age of nine. He continued to have emotional and interpersonal difficulties after his hospitalization, often exhibiting intense fear of abandonment when staff refused his minor requests. He often misinterpreted others' intentions as malevolent and exhibited symptoms of complex post-traumatic stress disorder (C-PTSD), including difficulty falling asleep, emotional dysregulation, dissociation, hyper/hypo-arousal, somatosensory deprivation, interpersonal instability, a belief that he was a "bad child", and occasional self-harming behaviour.

About the medical team

A treatment team was assembled to support Taro's therapy and overall environment from a trauma-informed perspective. The team included a clinical psychologist as the MBT therapist, a primary child psychiatrist, a primary nurse, an occupational therapist, a social worker, and a teacher. As part of his treatment, we agreed that Taro should meet individually with a therapist, based on the time-limited MBT model of working with children (Midgley et al., 2017; Juffermans & Muller, 2020). The progress of therapy was shared at morning check-ins and weekly conferences, and regular updates were provided on Taro's behaviour, mental state and support needs. The work began, however, with an assessment period, where, the MBT therapist, tried to develop a "mentalizing profile" of Taro, including how he was doing in terms of the "building blocks" of mentalizing – i.e. his capacity for attention control, affect regulation and explicit mentalizing (Midgley et al., 2017; Verheugt-Pleiter & Zevalkink, 2021).

On the cultural differences in emotional expression when translating Japanese conversations into English

Translating the therapeutic interaction between the child and the therapist from Japanese into English sometimes loses delicate yet critical nuances. When expressing emotions in Japanese, the "subjects" and "objects" are often omitted. Instead of stating who felt an emotion (e.g., "You are nervous"), Japanese uses more vague emotional expressions such as "Kincho-surune" ("there's some tense-feeling" or "might there be some nervousness"), which articulates the presence of an emotion without attributing it to a specific individual. This allows the therapist and child to share the same emotional space, even though each person may have a different kind of engagement with that feeling.

In translating my conversations with Taro into English, I've noticed that I consciously (sometimes pre-consciously) differentiate between using or omitting "subjects" when expressing emotions that arose during the therapy. The direct English translation does not clearly reflect the fact that subjects (i.e., who was feeling an emotion) were often consciously omitted in situations where implicit emotional attunement was more crucial, or during emotionally charged situations. For Japanese people, explicit communication of who is feeling the emotion can sometimes feel invasive. Placing the emotion "between individuals" in "places" or in "landscapes", without using a subject, provides a safer environment for processing emotions. It's as if the emotions become a shared landscape which the child and therapist can explore together. I think this aspect of the Japanese language makes it a uniquely effective tool for MBT with children, in facilitating a more natural and inter-subjective experience of shared emotions between therapist and child.

Therapy assessment phase: epistemic hypervigilance, pretend mode

The first time Taro came into the therapy room, he seemed fine and unconcerned. However, I (the MBT therapist) noticed his smile was awkward, his body seemed stiff and strained, and he lacked body awareness, as evidenced by wearing a long-sleeved jacket despite the heat. He was restless, reacted to the slightest noises, smells and fluorescent lights, and was startled by the sound of doors closing.

I felt Taro's nervousness, and realized that I had become similarly tense, breathing shallowly. So I first tried to regulate my own breathing to relax, as I thought it is important for the therapist to be aware of my own physical sensations and emotions first, when I meet clients who are not very aware of their physical sensations. Then I asked Taro in a calm tone, "there's some tense-feeling ...?" Taro tilted his head and said, "Don't know ..." Keeping a calm tone and speaking slowly while observing his reactions, I replied "Okay... since it's quite usual there's often a sense of tense-feeling in an unfamiliar environment with strangers. Don't you think?" Then he said, "yeah ... maybe".

After putting into words something about the emotional temperature in this way, I introduced myself, asked Taro what he liked to do and what he was good at. Taro told me that he liked sports and muscle training. I attempted to create a warm space and be responsive, but Taro's attention seemed to be somewhere else, and I found it difficult to feel an emotional connection with him. A bit later on I invited Taro to play the animal figure image game in an effort to make the atmosphere more playful. It's a game where you and your partner pick animal figures that you think resemble each other, then try to guess why you each chose those animals. Taro chose a "lion" as his self-image. I guessed the reason why he chose it and asked him, "Did you choose the lion because you want to become strong?" Taro said in a dissatisfied tone, "No, it's because *I am strong*, like a lion. I don't know why, but I always think about being strong." I realized my misunderstandings and validated that being strong was important to Taro. Then I asked him to choose an animal to represent me. He chose a shark, explaining that "[you're] a bit scary", while using the shark in his hands to attack the lion. For the most important person in his life, he chose a whale shark, saying "It's my mum. I want her to be calm and peaceful."

For my own self-image, I told Taro that I was like a cow because I like to take things slowly. When we shared that we had very different images and thoughts from each other, Taro seemed interested. Next, he suggested hiding the figures and letting me find them. I noticed Taro's curiosity and desire to play with others, despite his fear of engaging.

Difficulties with attention control and emotional regulation

In the following three assessment sessions Taro seemed restless, picking up different things and playing with them, but not for long. He seemed to want to do something but was hesitant. I gently asked him, "Is there anything you would like to try?" He said, "Don't know." I then noticed his shoulders were tense and asked him whether he was feeling anything in his body. At first Taro said, "Don't know." I looked at him with a slightly curious look on my face. After a brief pause, he continued: "Um, well, but maybe a bit scared ..." I asked him what he was scared of. He said, "Don't know ... but [I] feel like [you're] going to bite me ... since [you're] looking at me and asking [me] a lot of questions ..." Briefly taken aback, I thanked him for sharing his fear with me and apologized for unintentionally scaring him by looking at him and asking questions. I explained that I was just curious to get to know him better.

Taro then found a toy gun with sponge bullets, picked it up and started shooting wildly. As the bullets grazed me, I said to Taro, "Wow, that's scary." I wondered if my questions or my gaze felt like bullets being fired at him. He had difficulty controlling his attention, so I suggested creating a "target" and shooting at it so we could both feel safe in this small room. I also encouraged him to focus on the target (attention control). At first, he couldn't hit the target at all and became irritated. I gave him encouraging words, like "Nice control!" or "Relax your arms and look at the target" to promote awareness of the state of his body. Taro got gradually better at hitting the target and appeared modestly pleased with his performance. I mirrored and amplified his joy by proclaiming "Yeah! You made it!" with a smile.

In this phase, attention was paid to regulating his arousal levels. I also tried to safely promote Taro's attentional control in a playful and safe manner. I tried to set limits and boundaries through play and communication so that he could experience feeling safe with others despite the presence of internal fear and anger.

In the next session, Taro said he wanted to draw a picture, but he froze in front of the paper. I thought my curiosity might be frightening him, so I pretended to look away. Taro quickly drew a separated convex and concave shape and two snakes, hiding the image from my view with his arms. I gently asked him about the snakes. Taro said that one snake was the ruler of the dark world of the dead, and the other snake was controlled by the dark snake, sometimes doing bad things without meaning to. I said it was an interesting story and that I'd like to hear more about it. But Taro put the drawing away, saying that he couldn't think of anything else and that he was bored.

Taro often seemed disconnected from his mind when a feeling was starting to emerge. I tried to warmly mirror these subtle changes in his facial/physical expression when they occurred, because I sensed his fear there. "Marked mirroring" through gentle facial expressions and soft tones was my attempt to suggest that he might be feeling something there, without being invasive, and to implicitly convey the message that it was okay to feel it. I would then sometimes carefully inquired if something was happening inside him. I was also aware that my curiosity may be threatening to him, so I tried to maintain a safe space as well as communicate and attune in more implicit ways.

Summary of the assessment phase

It appeared that Taro was in epistemic hypervigilance during most of the assessment meetings, with strong physical tension (embodiment of trauma) and difficulties in emotional regulation and attentional control. His mentalizing was underdeveloped and he often seemed to be in "pretend mode" (e.g. when he said "I am strong like a lion!"). The need for strength also seemed to cause a preoccupation with physical masculinity, which could have sexual connotations. I felt that a strong need for attachment might underlie his over-adaptation. At the same time, however, I sensed a vital spark in Taro, a love of physical movement, a sense of curiosity about others and an ability to play. This gave me hope for his future.

In the time-limited MBT model, the assessment ends with a focus formulation, which helps to provide a shared focus for the work. Using the Lion as a metaphor, I suggested a focus formulation for Taro, and then the medical team: "What does 'strength' mean for this lion? Let's go on a journey together to discover what it takes to strengthen his emotional muscles." After sharing this with Taro, the therapist then discussed the assessment with the medical team, including the following points of concern for Taro's future treatment:

- Risk assessment for Taro's self-harming behaviour and possible future treatment concerns.
- Monitoring difficult feelings that may arise for the therapist and the medical team.
- Checking that the therapist's own mentalization was online.
- Maintaining a "not knowing" stance to be open and curious.
- That genuine emotional warmth will be the key to building epistemic trust.

We also agreed that maintaining "we-mode" (Asen & Fonagy, 2021; Bevington et al., 2017) within the medical team was crucial to achieving these goals.

The beginning phase: building a relationship, epistemic trust and stimulating post-traumatic play

Post-traumatic play and the therapist's non-mentalizing

In the ensuing sessions, Taro started playing with monster figures in a sandbox. He became quite absorbed, putting the monsters against each other in battle, stating they were mortal enemies. Over time, the enemies got mixed up and Taro started making everyone kill each other. Sometimes, he would give one of the figures god-like powers and pretend it was saving his allies. But "the god" always ended up betraying and dominating. I tried to mentalize the situations explicitly and create a short story, but he ignored my comments and the world became more aggressive and chaotic.

When I shared my thoughts about what was happening in the sandbox with the monsters, Taro suddenly picked up a toy gun, pointed it at me and said, "Bang! [You're] dead!". He then pointed the gun at his own head, then pretended to shoot himself and fall over dead. After that, Taro initiated a very dominant, post-traumatic play which prevented me from intervening. During this play, Taro harshly told me that, "You're buried and trapped in the grave! no one will hear you, no matter how much you scream!". He then suddenly changed his attitude and gently said "It's lonely here, isn't it?", and offered me a piece of bread. He continued, "Now I'll show you a dream from the past."

He acted out a scene involving "parents fighting and abusing their child" and added that "someone touched the child's private parts, but the parents pretended that no one had touched the child".

His acting was so realistic, and I felt scared and stuck. Seeing that I was overwhelmed, Taro said, "Now I'm going to take you to the other world." In this imaginary journey, Taro next took me to "heaven", where the child had kind parents and siblings, and received lots of treats and toys. In this "heaven" world, the characters spoke in a suspiciously unrealistic manner. Realizing that I was uncomfortable, Taro became irritated and desperate – "Would you rather be in heaven or in the grave? Choose one or the other! *Now!*" This transpired so rapidly that I became overwhelmed and fell into a non-mentalizing state. Having to choose one or the other felt intensely uncomfortable, but I also felt pressure to give him a "correct" answer. "It's really hard to choose one or the other. I want to go back to the world outside the grave with you." Taro was clearly disappointed and replied, "[I] don't want to play such a lonely game anymore …"

After this intense session, I gathered the team for a discussion. With the warm reflections and support of the doctor and other team members, we arrived at a few conclusions: Firstly, given his exposure to various forms of violence from an early age, it was understandable that Taro would show confusion about right and wrong, sexual confusion and fear, as well as despair and dissociation. Taro, who seemed to view himself as a ghostly, powerless child, may have been feeling a sense of urgency to choose between one of two extremes: remained in despair and loneliness in the grave, or fantasize about a dissociated world full of omnipotent beings. During the post-traumatic play, I vicariously experienced Taro's deep suffering, pain, and loneliness. I realized that I had fallen into a teleological mode of thinking: "I have to save and protect this child by giving him the *right* answer." I also considered the possibility that Taro was uncertain whether I would notice the depth of his loneliness or whether I would be just a passing stranger "giving him a piece of bread".

In the next session, Taro started playing with the monster figures again. He brought the monster figure in his hand close to the zombie figure he had placed in my hand. Then he shoved the fang-like tentacles of his monster into the zombie's mouth. In a fake zombie voice, I pleaded, "Oh, please help, it's scary!", but Taro didn't seem to hear me and continued to violently stab the zombie with a blank dissociative face. I called Taro's name again. Startled, he replied "Oh, what? … Did something happen?" Then he whispered to me, "you should pretend you didn't see anything". I carefully responded, "When something scary like this happens, it's natural to want to pretend it never happened." He promptly shouted, "Don't say a word!" After a moment of silence, I explained how experiences like this can be scary, uncomfortable, and unbearable, not only for the zombie but for anyone, including me. I asked if he had ever experienced such feelings before. Turning his back to me, he replied "maybe …" I told Taro that being forced to do something you don't want to do, or being forced to accept something physically unpleasant, can leave an incredibly deep scar on one's heart, and such scars are sometimes related to our past experiences.

Listening in silence, Taro asked me in a depressed voice, "So you mean if someone does something bad, they have to 'confess' everything, right?" "Bad things?", I gently asked with a surprised look on my face, since the conversation had taken an unexpected turn. "Don't want to talk about that", Taro replied. I decided to press further, "What does 'confession' mean?" Taro responded, "Don't know … someone said that a long time ago." I asked if we could pause and think about this a bit more, adding, "I'm sorry if I made you feel confused. And I was a little confused too. So I want to ask you, since I am a bit worried about whether you think you had done something wrong and you feel you need to 'confess' about?" Taro nodded. There was a long period of silence. Then I asked, "I wonder if you think you're here because you've done something wrong?" Taro nodded again in agreement. I explained that he was here to be cared for, not to confess or be punished. I followed up with, "When things are so unbearable, people naturally become confused about what's good and what's bad. It's not your fault." Taro covered his face with his jacket and collapsed onto the sofa. I reassured him that together we can find a way to feel safe here. I also mentioned that he could ask or talk about anything with the team members.

In the team discussion, we conjectured that in an institutional environment the emotional care from adults was insufficient. Thus, sexual contact was a frighteningly invasive experience for him, but at the same time, repeating it with the children may have been the only way for Taro to find warmth, softness, and a momentary sense of security and connection. We also considered how we could convey to Taro that all children should be cared for and protected first, rather than being blamed or held responsible for issues beyond their control.

Emotional regulation via martial arts training

In the following session, Taro asked me to practise wrestling with him. I considered that Taro may have wanted to confirm that he had the power in our relationship, and that an unconscious desire for sexual contact was also at play. As Taro had recently become interested in martial arts, I suggested karate instead. The movement of karate is based on traditional *kata* (form), which requires awareness, concentration, body and breath control. Practising karate also seemed like an ideal way for Taro to safely release his aggression. Taro readily agreed, so I invited him to practise standing while concentrating on *tanden* (the lower dantian) where energy is said to be concentrated. I explained that noticing his physical sensations was very important. If he could share what he noticed about his body and mind, that would also be helpful for me. We watched short karate videos together on an iPad (joint attention) to learn how to do a kumite (pretend sparring where you stop just before making contact with your partner) and kata (patterns of movement or positions practised either alone or in pairs). We practised coordinated breathing and movement, counting out "one, two, three!". At first it was difficult to get in sync. Taro and I looked at each other and laughed about how our timing didn't work out. Taro was a quick learner and seemed to enjoy the sensation of moderating his strength so as not to hurt me. Through these interactions I began to feel an emotional connection with Taro.

Existential questions

In a later session, Taro asked me if I had ever had a child, and what it was like to have a child. When I gently asked him why he was interested, he replied "No, it's nothing. Never mind." and stopped the conversation. Taro seemed to shut down whenever questions were directed at him. I wondered about the intent of his original question (about my experience with bearing children). For Taro, turning his attention to his early life might be a sign that he was trying to get in touch with the meaning of his birth, and of his own existence. He repeated the same question in our next session. With as much warmth and sincerity as I could muster, I explained that I had the experience of giving birth to children. I added that, "I think giving birth was a very, very special event in life, and probably for you and your mom as well." Taro listened intently. I wanted to tell him that he was not alone at the moment of his birth, adding "The moment of birth is a collaborative process between the baby and the mother." Instead of responding directly, Taro asked if he could bring his life story workbook to our next therapy session. I welcomed it.

In our next session, Taro brought his life story workbook, which his former social worker had created for him. While looking at the family genogram together, he mentioned that he hadn't seen his mother for a long time, and he had never seen his father. He also talked about moving from one institution to another, and how the people caring for him eventually changed or left. "They said I would see my mom again someday, but I haven't seen her for years. I don't know if the adults are telling me the truth." I reassured him that the medical staff and I were thinking about him, that he could express his thoughts and ask questions about his life, and that if he wanted, his opinions would be shared with the team and the conversation about Taro would be discussed openly.

Middle phase: fear of abandonment and trying to hold Taro's mind in mind

While I was away on a business trip for a week, a nurse who had been taking care of Taro resigned suddenly. Taro became emotionally unstable and failed to show up for his next scheduled session with me. Another nurse informed me that Taro was upset and panicking because the in-hospital class seasonal event in the ward had prevented him from heading to the therapy session on time.

When I arrived at the ward, Taro was in the corridor crying and shouting. A doctor was holding Taro's hand and speaking quietly to him to calm him down. I sat down next to Taro and waited for him to relax. While Taro was crying, I wondered what was going on in his mind. After he calmed down a bit and hung his head in despair, I murmured my thoughts into words, as if questioning myself but loud enough that he could hear it. When I murmured whether he feared that our whole relationship would be over because he was late for therapy, Taro nodded slightly. Here I thought that Taro was in a psychic equivalent mode triggered by abandonment anxiety, where not being able to physically see the therapist or being late for the therapy would make him fear losing the relationship with others. So I first validated his deep fear and emotional wounds, and reassured him that I think about him even when we don't see each other. After he regained his composure, I also told him that I wouldn't end his therapy or disappear without explanation just for being late or absent, so as to explicitly convey that I was predictable and available for him. Taro listened intently, but seemed reluctant and said he didn't want to come to the therapy. I decided to respect his opinion and wait a while, thinking that the experience of being accepted in the way he was would be important to Taro.

After a period of resistance and a cancellation, Taro returned to the therapy. During the session, he looked out the window and asked, "What would you do if I fell out of the window?" With a concerned look, I explained that I'd help him right away. He looked relieved for just a moment. A little while later, I mentioned that I had heard about the nurse suddenly quitting. The fear and loneliness triggered by that event might have led Taro to be anxious about whether I could truly support him when he needed help. He laid silently on the sofa and covered his face for a long time. I felt sadness radiating from his body and watched him in silence. The silence was broken by Taro's sudden, loud passing of gas. We immediately looked at each other in surprise, then burst out laughing. I joked with him that it is important to "let the bad gases" out sometimes.

At the end of the session, Taro came up with the idea of making a promissory note: we would write our names on a piece of paper, then cut it in half. In the next session, we would both bring the piece of paper with our name on it and stick them back together again. In subsequent sessions, a ritual emerged: Taro would tell me what he wanted me to remember, what he needed me to prepare for the next week, and assigned a bit of homework to me. In the following session, he would check if I had honoured our promises and done my homework. I also began taking photos of the artwork he created in the therapy, as well as photos of himself, and created a special album just for him.

Considering Taro's condition in therapy, the team members tried to engage Taro more frequently, expressing empathy for how hard it must have been that his favourite nurse had left him, and that it wasn't his fault – just the nurse's private decision. At the beginning of the therapy, the staff members and myself often struggled to remember what Taro wanted from us, and Taro frequently insinuated that he was not being cared for. Taro's cry for help and outpouring of fear and pain at being abandoned, along with our effort to "hold his mind in mind", allowed Taro to gradually be present in my mind. In parallel, Taro's mind was becoming more capable of stably holding the therapist's presence, as well.

Creating a secret shelter

In the next session, at Taro's request, I prepared some cardboard boxes. Taro was delighted and enthusiastically built his own "secret shelter". The shelter was shaped like an igloo with a spacious room at the end of a narrow tunnel. I thought it resembled a womb. He put a blanket inside, curled up and laid down. "I like it here ... even though it's not the ideal shape", he said. "I can sleep here ... I mean, I want to stay here forever ..." Taro tapped on the inside of the shelter with his finger to make a sound. In turn, I tapped on the same spot from the outside, using the same rhythm. We played this rhythm tap game for a while. Then Taro sang a song he used to listen to at his former institution (the lyrics are "There is so much in this world I don't know"). He began to talk about past memories – what the room in his previous orphanage looked like, and some of the fragmented episodes which occurred there. His memories generated pictures in my mind. Then he shifted to the memories of his mother. "She was crying when I was taken to the children's home." I asked what he felt at the time. Taro replied, "I was sad." I nodded deeply with understanding. I asked what Taro thought his mother was thinking at that time. "I think she was sad too", he guessed. He subsequently remembered that she was always angry with him when he was little, but he didn't understand why. His memories were quite fragmented. At this point, his posture began to slump and he started to yawn. I sensed that his arousal level was dropping, so I paused the conversation and invited him to slow down the pace of the play, move his body slowly to help him coming back into his window of tolerance.

Self-injury and need for care

In the following session, Taro confessed that he had been frustrated and punched a wall, injuring himself. He insisted that it wasn't that painful. He took the bandage off and showed me his self-inflicted wound. He laid on the sofa and covered his face again, exclaiming, "I'm exhausted ..." Soon after, Taro said, "You know what? The moment I got hurt, I didn't really feel anything – I was laughing instead!" I explained that sometimes when a person is hurt or in shock, the mind shuts down to protect them from feeling anything painful. Taro responded, "I know. I saw it in a movie before. A guy saw a ghost and fell down with a big smile on his face." Then Taro began to sing a song, "you need sunshine for your frozen heart". I commented that a frozen heart indeed needs the kind of warmth provided by sunshine.

It was clear that Taro felt alone with the heavy burdens in his heart. I held out my palms and asked Taro to put his hands on top of mine and put his weight on them. Taro was a little shy, but he did as I asked. I told him I could feel him, and that he could rest his heavy emotional burden on me, just like he was doing physically with his hands right now. He responded shyly, "I'm not sure if I can do that", while applying more weight on my hands. This activity helped Taro gradually gain a sense of security through touch. On one occasion, I put my hand on his back (with his permission) when he was lying down in a state of sadness and depression and asked how it felt. Taro replied, "My back feels warm", then closed his eyes and seemed to be relieved.

I shared this episode with the team. Taro required sleeping medication in order to sleep, but from this point on the nurses began a new routine: at bedtime, they would ask where his body was tired, then try some relaxing exercises with him. Sometimes they put their hands on Taro's back, at his request. Taro began to fall asleep more smoothly with the reassuring touch of the nurses.

Walk in the forest: shared wonder and an existential question

It was a pleasant autumn day, and Taro had been wanting to leave the hospital for a while. So, I got permission to take him for a walk. We went to a nearby forest with a small shrine. I suggested we look for something beautiful in the forest. Taro's reply was less than enthusiastic: "I've never thought of anything as beautiful before." I picked up some fallen berries and smelled them, then invited Taro to do the same. After a brief hesitation, Taro nervously moved his face closer then sniffed the berries. "Oh, I see what you mean!" He began collecting fallen leaves, asking, "Is this beautiful?" I put the question back to Taro: "What do you think?" Taro replied, "I think it's beautiful." I told him I thought so, too. We enjoyed the coolness of the forest air, the smell of the trees and the sound of falling leaves. Surrounded by nature, we strolled aimlessly, noting various sensations that we both were experiencing. Taro hugged a big tree in the pathway to the shrine and said, "feels good". We paused at the shrine and each clapped our hands together and made a wish. Taro told me that his prayer was a secret.

During the approach to the shrine, Taro found a large seed lying in the path. In Japanese culture, the pathway to a shrine symbolizes the birth canal and the shrine itself represents the womb. I was moved by the way Taro gently held the seed in the palm of his hand, as if he was protecting a foetus. He said he wanted to plant the seed and let it grow, see what kind of flowers would bloom. Falling into doubt again, Taro hedged, "But … it's probably just a weed. I don't want to get my hopes up, because if I get my hopes up too high, I'll be disappointed."

Returning back to the hospital for the end of our session, we watched the sunset together from the rooftop floor. Quietly watching the sun set, I felt as if we were being embraced by nature, bathed in an orange glow. I felt a deep sense of nostalgia, like I had seen this landscape at some point in the past. We sat in silence for a while longer. In the silence, Taro quietly murmured, "I wonder why I was born …"

His words seemed to dissolve into the scenery. I tried to understand his feeling and the meaning of his question about being, from his perspective. Soon I stopped consciously thinking, opened up my senses and let myself absentmindedly surrender to the present moment, to which no words or concepts could be attached. It was an oceanic feeling, and I felt a deep sense of connection with Taro, and all things around us.

I think this unforgettable feeling was a kind of spirituality deeply connected to the everyday life of the Japanese, known as *mono no aware*. It was a feeling similar to empathy but different from the Western concept of "empathy", which is based on the clear distinction between self and other. Instead, it was a feeling of accepting impermanence of all things with "a sensitivity of human emotion to all things, in which there is no distinction between self and other, things and creatures, between ourselves and the cosmos" (Togashi, 2024).

I felt that Taro's question – "I wonder why I was born?" – did not have a "right" answer. Instead, I chose to share the honest feelings which came to mind: "This was such a beautiful moment to have shared with you, and I am glad to have met you. Thank you for being born."

Mentalizing the relation and building the narrative of his life

Taro gradually expressed more interest in engaging in activities he was proficient at or enjoyed. But he frequently gave up prematurely in disappointment, saying "Anyway, it's impossible." I wondered if Taro perhaps struggled with expecting too much. I told him that he was courageous to try something new even when he feels a mix of both high expectations and a sense of resignation. Taro sighed, a sceptical look on his face. At this moment, I decided to explicitly mentalize the relationship between us: "I get the impression that you sometimes feel disappointed in me that I don't live up to your expectations, and that sometimes you find it hard to believe what I say?" Taro nodded, indicating this was accurate.

I mentioned that there were several moments in our last few sessions when he suddenly went quiet or fell into a bad mood. Further, when I asked what happened he was unwilling to answer. So I asked him to recall what was going on in his mind during those silent or bad mood moments. Taro simply replied, "Don't know …" Then he clarified a bit without using the "subject": "Even if I knew what [I was] thinking, [I] didn't want to tell [you] because I knew it would make [you] sad." I was surprised and asked what he meant. He said he knew that I would have negative feelings towards him if he told me how he really felt. I validated him by saying, "It's natural [for you] to be concerned about sharing your honest thoughts, but I'd like to hear how you feel. I believe our relationship has been strengthened by telling each other how we feel." Taro explained that in the past, when he had told adults how he really felt, he had only been attacked, ignored, or cast away. After pausing to think a bit more, he added, "I did a lot of terrible things here, but you and the doctor did not abandon me." I nodded and told him, "If you feel that way, I think we can play a new game: the 'sharing honest feelings' game."

Over time, Taro began to share feelings that he wished he could have expressed to his mother. He talked about the anger and sadness from not understanding why she had never come to see him, why she had frequently neglected him, and why she left him when he was just a baby.

Taro also began to express his dissatisfaction with me as well. He said that sometimes he didn't like the way I talked to him and suspected that I lied to keep him happy. He also said he was disappointed and embarrassed when I failed at something. He also believed that "normal" people might think he was "weird". If I didn't think he was weird, then I was perhaps not normal. I confessed that I'm not perfect at all and make a lot of mistakes. I said that it's quite natural for Taro to feel bad and ashamed about my lack of perfection. I also apologized for my mistakes and misunderstandings, and praised the fact that he chose to speak honestly and non-violently about his concerns.

Taro sighed, saying he still couldn't believe that what I had said was true. He suspected that I was just pretending to accept him. I reflected on my own feelings and behaviour and told Taro that my acceptance of him was genuine. Taro doubted my sincerity, saying "that's an absolute lie", then laid down on the sofa with his jacket over his head. After a long silence, he peeked out from under his jacket with a grim expression and asked me, "Really? Really? Really?" I replied using the same rhythm, "Really, really, really." He shook his head and asked again, "Really? Really? Really?" We repeated this exchange over and over. I sensed that we had arrived at a critical moment in the "telling each other how we really feel" game, so I looked Taro in the eye and firmly said, "Really" with all my heart.

Taro paused and stared at my eyes for a while. He seemed to be thinking about something. Then he simply nodded three times, without words. He started to laugh, and I couldn't help laughing along with him. At the end of the session, Taro confided, "I had been fearing that I was actually alone all this time, but trying my best not to feel it. But the truth is, my mind was in tears the whole time." I validated Taro's fear and sadness, acknowledging that he had endured very difficult emotions on his own for a long time. Then I thanked him for sharing his honest feelings with me.

Increased assertiveness and the importance of being held in others' minds

From the next session onwards, Taro began actively asking those around him about his future "When can I leave the hospital?", "Will I ever see my mother again?", etc. He started expressing his own wishes and concerns, and his new awareness of his anxiety allowed him to begin dealing with it proactively e.g., taking a time out, talking to people instead of waiting for his emotions to explode, etc. We also worked on anger management and social skills through activities such as writing the feelings of the characters in speech bubbles.

He talked about his desire to be discharged from the hospital and live a more normal life, either in a new institution or with a foster family. On the other hand, Taro was concerned about his treatment ending once he was discharged from hospital. I told him that the doctor, the team, and I were proud of his willingness to embrace a new life and that we would continue to support him. Meanwhile, the medical team and I discussed Taro's concerns and the practical difficulties he might face in his new life. Before therapy, Taro made frequent complaints to the hospital staff, but now he was sharing more positive experiences with hospital staff. Even more impressive, he proudly shared that he had demonstrated karate at a hospital event and received a round of applause.

Ending phase: forgetting, remembering, exchanging treasures and letters, holding mind in mind

After the dates were set for Taro's discharge and admission to another facility, I spoke with Taro about ending his therapy. He replied, "Part of me is happy to get out of here, but another part of me doesn't want to end therapy. I'm not sure if I'll be able to manage on my own." I reassured him that it's perfectly normal to be anxious about moving to a new environment. At the same time, I told Taro that the team and I believe he has the strength to do well in his new environment. Taro responded, "Time flies ... Can you imagine what I will be like when I grow up? Won't you forget about me?" I told Taro I would never forget about him, and he will always be in my heart. A little while later, Taro and I looked through the photo albums and calendars from our therapy sessions. Taro suggested we make some kind of memorial "treasure" or "charm" together and exchange them, so we could hold each other's mind in mind. I told Taro that was a fantastic idea.

In the final session, we exchanged our treasures to hold each other's mind in mind: linking back to the focus formulation from the start of our work together, I gave Taro a letter and a key chain with a lion emblazoned on it, and Taro gave me a handmade friendship bracelet. Taro said, "I'm so sad…" I replied softly, "I'm really sad, too." We silently shared the weight of our sadness and the unspoken feelings tied to our farewell. Then I shared my reflection on Taro's growth, specifically that he had become stronger in mind as well as body, that he can tell others what he is feeling and thinking, and he can value his vulnerabilities. Taro had tears in his eyes. I reassured him that he will always be in my heart.

To me, the journey together with "Taro the lion" was sometimes like an exploration in the forest or diving into the depths of the ocean together. In my letter to Taro, I wrote that the time we spent together was profoundly memorable and precious. I also mentioned that he had his own unique and precious "lion's heart" deep within his heart. This lion's heart represents his sensitive heart, curiosity, willingness to take on challenges, and ability to connect with others through his interests and strengths. I encouraged him to cherish that "lion's heart". At the end of the letter, I wrote that finding and trusting someone who genuinely cares will give him the strength to rely on others in times of need.

Regarding Taro's discharge, the medical team and I worked on a detailed information-sharing and handover process with the new facility and school. A few months later we received a letter and photo from the facility saying that Taro was doing well. The photo was taken in a restaurant with the facility staff, and Taro was holding a cup with a picture of a lion on it. The medical team and I were surprised and delighted. It might have been just a coincidence, but we certainly felt a connection with Taro, and sensed that what we shared and built during therapy seemed to live further in Taro, and he was developing further with this felt connection inside him.

Acknowledgements

In writing this chapter, I would like to express my sincere gratitude to the children and my colleagues, who taught me so much. Above all to Nicole Muller, who always guided me with insightful comments and warm validation.

Note

1 This is a fictional case combining elements from multiple real-life cases that share similarities.

References

Asen, E. & Fonagy, P. (2021). *Mentalization-based treatment with families*. Guilford Press.
Bevington, D., Fuggle, P., Cracknell, L., Fonagy, P. (2017). *Adaptive mentalization-based integrative treatment: A guide for teams to develop systems of care*. Oxford University Press. doi:10.1093/med-psych/9780198718673.001.0001.
Juffermans, M. & Muller, N. (2020). Case-study: Mentalization-based treatment, a time-limited approach, for a boy with a mild intellectual disability and trauma. *Global Journal of Intellectual & Developmental Disabilities*, 7(2). doi:10.19080/gjidd.2020.07.555706.

Midgley, N., Ensink, K., Lindqvist, K., Malberg, N., & Muller, N. (2017). *Mentalization-based treatment for children: A time-limited approach*. American Psychological Association. doi:10.1037/0000028-000.

Togashi, K. (2024). Seeing psychoanalytic culture from an Asian perspective. Paper presented at Pre-Conference of IAPSP 45th Annual International Conference, "Tragic Person Today: Existence and Meaning in Life and Clinical Practice", Rome, Italy, 24 October.

Verheugt-Pleiter, A. & Zevalkink, J. (2021). *Mentalizing in child therapy: Guidelines for clinical practitioners*, 2nd edition. Routledge. doi:10.4324/9781003167242.

Chapter 6

Working with school-age children (II)

The case of Pamir

Sibel Halfon, Hazal Çelik and Dilara Güvenç

Pamir was a 9-year-old boy who received therapy in time-limited mentaliza-tion-based treatment for children (MBT-C) at Istanbul Bilgi University Psy-chotherapy Centre (IBUPC), which is the only low-fee sliding scale community outpatient clinic in Turkey that conducts psychodynamic and mentalization-based therapy with children. The clinic is a training, research and psychotherapy centre. It is the primary practicum site for clinical psy-chology master's-level students at Istanbul Bilgi University, who practice psychodynamic and mentalization-based therapy with children under the clinical supervision of experienced practitioners in the field.

When first referred, Pamir presented with a high degree of epistemic vigi-lance, a common feature in children who have experienced trauma – and a feature which provides challenges to therapy. As we hope to show, the core features of a mentalizing stance, that is, genuine curiosity towards the child's mind and empathic attunement, were essential to help this child feel safe and recognized in the therapist's mind. Moreover, due to the developmental trau-mas he had experienced, he had an underdeveloped capacity for mentaliza-tion. In this chapter we will explore how attention-control interventions, which aimed to identify internal states and link them to intentions in the outside world, were essential to help build agency and self-awareness. We will also show how the therapist attended closely to escalating emotions in the sessions and used empathetic validation to help regulate the child's heightened states of arousal.

In what follows we will present Pamir's therapy to illustrate the time-lim-ited MBT-C model employed at our clinic. The therapy was provided as part of a randomized clinical trial (RCT) of MBT-C that our centre was carrying out.[1] During the RCT, every child and parent had a total of 15 sessions, out of which three sessions were designated for assessment purposes. The assess-ment sessions, which were conducted jointly by the child therapist and the parent-worker, aimed to build a mentalizing profile of the children and their parents that can be used for treatment planning. Furthermore, each child received an attachment-based story stem evaluation (Bretherton et al., 1990) and the Child Attachment Interview (CAI; Target et al., 2003), providing a

DOI: 10.4324/9781032713441-10

comprehensive understanding of their attachment schemas and mentalization abilities. At the end of the assessment phase, a focus formulation was presented that captured a component of the child's central experiences in the form of a story or a metaphor. This aimed to communicate to the family that the therapist strived to create meaning around the child's problems while engaging the family in the process. After this, the child and parents were seen separately by their respective therapists, with a joint review session at the mid-point.

Reason for referral

Pamir[2] was referred for therapy due to conflicts with his mother and difficulties at school. Pamir's mother reported constant fights at home, particularly regarding Pamir's responsibilities, such as completing his homework or doing his house chores in a timely fashion. When Pamir failed to complete these, they got into severe fights, and the mother reported feeling very impatient and angry at him. In order to control herself, she had to distance herself from him, and she admitted to hitting him a few times. Alongside these difficulties at home, Pamir struggled with his academic work, had very few friends, and experienced severe physical bullying from his peers.

Pamir's developmental history

During the pregnancy, Pamir's parents separated due to the father's severe physical abuse towards the mother, leading to their break-up and permanent estrangement. As a result, Pamir has never had the chance to meet his father. His mother stated how her relationship with Pamir was a source of comfort from the difficulties she faced with her husband during her pregnancy: "I always wanted to have a son. Whenever I argued with my husband, I spoke with Pamir; I spoke to my belly." A severe physical fight between the parents at 33 weeks into the pregnancy triggered the mother's premature labour. Pamir had to be in the intensive care unit for 20 days due to lung problems. Every day, the mother visited the intensive care unit (ICU), but she could only breastfeed briefly with limited physical contact. Pamir could not develop the ability to suck. Nurses tried to improve the reflex by taping a pacifier to Pamir's mouth. Pamir used two pacifiers until age 2, one around his neck and the other in his mouth. He was described as a baby who slept a lot. At age 3, Pamir began to inquire about his father's identity and whereabouts, but his mother only provided limited information about their separation. He stopped asking questions afterward.

The mother had a very close relationship with Pamir. However, this closeness also involved a high degree of control on the mother's part, as she wanted Pamir to behave exactly how she wanted and follow her rules. As a result, Pamir mostly took on roles assigned by the mother and had to complete tasks beyond his developmental level. Pamir prepared his own breakfast, tidied the kitchen, and prepared for school by himself. During assessment sessions, the therapists were puzzled by this information because Pamir looked very clumsy and prone to accidents.

Initial family session and assessment

In the initial session, both the parent's and child's therapists were present to meet with Pamir and his mother. The goal of the session was to gain insight into the presenting problem and their interactions with each other.

Pamir entered the room, looked around and then sat on the chair looking down. He made very little eye contact with the therapists. He started to fidget with his hands and continued to look down. When asked to introduce himself, the therapists barely heard his voice. He was very focused on his body, playing with the fidget spinner toy he had brought. It seemed that he relied primarily on sensorimotor means to regulate himself. He barely responded to any of the therapists' questions and concentrated on small pieces of threads on his pants. When one therapist asked, "Do you know why you are here?", he said very quietly, "Because I fight", and then fell silent again.

The therapists changed their approach in the following assessment sessions and used play to communicate with the boy and his mother. They introduced an animal game, where each family member was asked to choose an animal that described themselves and other family members. This was a non-threatening way to engage with the family and gain a better understanding of their self- and other-representations. When the therapists inquired about the animal he had chosen for himself, Pamir silently displayed the cow. When asked why he chose the cow, he simply replied, "Because I like it." Pamir selected a lion for his mother, but when asked why, he shrugged and said he did not know. Later, he explained that he chose a lion because of his mother's hair. The therapists wondered (to themselves) whether the cow could represent a maternal role and possibly communicate a confusion of roles in the family. The lion, instead, brought to mind stronger and possibly more aggressive qualities.

From this initial encounter, it was evident that Pamir had difficulty describing his personality. He made no reference to mental states and was focused on physical attributes. A similar picture emerged in the Child Attachment Interview (CAI) administered before the therapy. When asked to pick three adjectives to describe himself, he responded, "I do not know", and upon further prompts, he said, "I am a good person", and "I am not a bad person". He could not come up with any specific instance or memory. Regarding his relationship with his mother, he said, "It is good to be with my mom", but could provide no specific descriptions. When his mother gets angry at him, he said, "Sometimes I go to my room and cry", but could not remember the last time this happened.

The only CAI question where Pamir provided a specific response was when asked if anything scared him. He mentioned a clown he watched on Netflix. He said, "I was so scared. So scared. Trying to run away. Scary. So bad. A noise comes. I am scared. The noise keeps coming. Scared." His attachment-based story stems were generally short, and all stories ended with the child feeling either bad about himself or scared. For example, in response to the "hurt knee story", he responded, "The child falls and his foot hurts. When they go to the hospital, they tell him that his foot will stay in a cast for a long time. He felt bad, scared that he had done something wrong."

First mentalization-based assessment session with Pamir

In the first assessment session conducted separately with Pamir, he came in and sat silently, gazing at the floor and slowly rocking in his chair. The therapist welcomed him warmly, trying to create a safe and supportive environment while at the same time noticing his reluctance to be present.

THERAPIST: Welcome … How does it feel to be here?

Pamir hesitated to respond.

THERAPIST: I have been thinking about you. About how it feels to be here.
PAMIR: I don't want to come.
THERAPIST: I noticed that sometimes it is very hard for you to be here. I wonder why you don't want to come.

Pamir stayed silent.

THERAPIST: You are free to say anything you want here.
PAMIR: I only want to come here when I want to.
THERAPIST: Oh, I see! That makes a lot of sense. You want to have a say in when you come.

In that initial encounter, the therapist validated Pamir's experience, implying that all parts of him (including the part of himself that did not want to be there) were welcome. She was curious to know about the child's mind and mirrored his need for agency. These qualities are at the heart of a mentalizing stance. Pamir started to feel more comfortable in the room after finding a warm and validating therapist. The therapist took this opportunity to show Pamir more about the room, and he noticed the Rubik's cube and started playing with it. The therapist joined him and started to play with the other Rubik's cube, communicating to the child non-verbally that they could find a way to be together in play. In the meantime, Pamir remembered his experience of the CAI and the story stem tasks:

PAMIR: I don't like questions. It is hard for me to answer questions about myself. I don't want to answer them.

THERAPIST: Yes, so many questions! It must have been so hard to go through that. It will be different here. We can do anything you like. Perhaps, you just want to play?

There was a shift in the child's attention in response to the therapist's remark. Being mentalized by the therapist ("it must have been hard") helped relax Pamir's epistemic vigilance. For the first time, he started to look around the room and noticed some of the toys. He held two swords and said, "You know they do it like this in video games?" (playing with the swords and showing the therapist how one protects oneself). The therapist embodied the same position and said, "Oh, yes, that is how you protect yourself." She kept the communication in play yet explicitly mentalized the need for protection, a theme pertinent for Pamir. They kept on playing with the swords.

Pamir's attachment and mentalization profile

At the end of this session, the two therapists came together to create the focus formulation, based on the mother's and child's attachment and mentalization profiles, their strengths and difficulties, and the early relational environment. Pamir's developmental history suggested severe disruptions in the early holding environment. The mother experienced a very difficult and traumatic pregnancy due to ongoing abuse from the father. Due to traumatic stress, the mother's ability to hold Pamir in mind as a separate individual was disrupted. The mother, with the support of her child and extended family, tried to stand strong against her traumas, and she was able to break up with the father. But despite this, Pamir was not "held" physically in the first few weeks after delivery and suffered from developmental problems.

The mother and Pamir were felt to have an enmeshed relationship that had disrupted Pamir's ability to develop a separate mind with his own desires and intentions. He had instead tried to conform to his mother's desires. He had difficulty identifying his feelings and describing his personality beyond physical and behavioural characteristics. His sense of self was pervaded by a sense of badness, fear, and hurt. Additionally, his attachment system was easily triggered, making it difficult for him to regulate himself. He relied on sensory and physical means for regulation. He mainly functioned in teleological mode, probably due to a lack of experience in having had his emotions mentalized, particularly painful and fearful ones. Despite these difficulties, Pamir was able to form a relationship with the therapist, who was curious about his mind and his feelings. Even though he was quite vigilant at first, Pamir felt more relaxed and trusting towards the end of the initial session. He also showed a capacity to communicate some of his intentions in play. These were all important strengths.

Viewing Pamir's relationship with his mother from a cultural perspective can shed light on certain aspects of their dynamic. Turkish society is collectivistic with some individualistic features (Sunar & Fişek, 2005). In collectivistic cultures, the " interdependent self-construal" places value on social harmony over expressing one's own internal states to promote group ideals and norms. Pamir's difficulty describing himself as a unique individual separate from his mother could also be a function of these cultural characteristics; however, it had been intensified due to the severe traumas of the dyad. Moreover, Pamir's mother's parenting involved a high level of authoritarian control, sometimes involving physical punishment. Even though this kind of parenting is common in Turkey, the therapists were required to assess the degree of risk, make a safety contract, and report to protective services if the physical violence continued. During the intake sessions, the therapists addressed this issue with the mother and made a safety contract to try and stop all physical punishment. They provided psycho-education on alternative discipline techniques that could promote self-control and positive regard.

The therapists also identified the following long-term aims for the therapy: Pamir, first and foremost, needed to feel safe both in his body and in interactions and to develop epistemic trust. He needed a therapeutic context where he felt understood and held in mind. The therapists felt that he would highly benefit from attention control and emotion regulation interventions that would enhance self/bodily awareness as well as regulate heightened states of arousal. Subsequently, the therapists aimed to incorporate these goals into a focus formulation that would be easily understood by both the child and the parent.

Focus formulation

In the focus formulation, which is shared with the family, the therapists wanted to highlight the challenges that the mother–child dyad had faced. They had to be extremely close to each other to protect themselves against the traumas, but at the same time, this closeness was hindering them. The therapists decided to use seashells to create a story to share. They set up the sand tray in the room and placed several seashells on it, then asked the mother and child to select one shell representing themselves.

THERAPIST: These seashells are living together at a beach, side by side. Can you imagine this beach Pamir?

PAMIR: There is a lot of sand there but not enough water.

THERAPIST: OK, these two seashells are living together at this beach with a lot of sand, but not enough water. They are very close to each other, with a strong tie. They try to protect themselves from the world around them. But they cannot really explore other places like other seas and beaches. Sometimes, these two seashells have fights, which becomes very difficult for them.

At this point in the story, the therapists were planning to introduce ways the dyad could feel safe so that they could explore the outside world, but Pamir wanted to continue the story. He said:

PAMIR: A big wave came and took them away. Towards the deep end. They get buried … Under the water. They are thinking about how to get out. The mother tries to get out. She comes out but can't find her son. The son is buried under. He is lost …Then he started telling another story:

PAMIR: Then there is a hill, and it collapses onto them. They lost their lives. They are stuck and cannot get out. Later on, an ambulance came to extract them, but they couldn't get out. [He brings an ambulance] Dadi-dadi … Once, we got stuck in the snow. I was very young. 4 or 5 years old. I was with my uncle. Come back! Help me.

The therapists recognized that this play showed traumatic qualities (Chazan et al., 2016). There were heightened levels of anxiety; the child was repeatedly expressing a traumatic sense of being lost and in danger, without any help coming for rescue. There was no resolution to the play narrative, instead it got disorganized and more overwhelming; and Pamir switched from talking about the characters in the third person ("they did this") to the first person ("I was very young"). The therapists decided to intervene to organize the play context to help him feel secure. When Pamir introduced an ambulance to rescue the seashells, the therapists actively intervened, rather than just following Pamir's play, and took the opportunity to revisit the focus formulation and come up with a therapy goal.

THERAPIST: These shells need a place to feel safe; they need strong protection. There are so many dangers in the world. The waves, the hills, the snow … We can help them find a shelter where they can feel safe.

Pamir was able to accept this active intervention and became a little more regulated. The therapists and the child then agreed that the metaphor of "finding a safe and secure shelter" would be the focus of the therapy.

Supervisory sessions

During Pamir's therapy, both therapists had weekly group supervision. The supervision played a crucial role in helping the therapists discuss their difficult emotions and challenges in maintaining a mentalizing stance. During the therapy sessions, Pamir's intense emotions often overwhelmed his therapist and made it difficult for her to mentalize Pamir. Pamir's play narrative was chaotic and disorganized, making the therapist question whether play-based interventions would effectively reach him. Moreover, Pamir's initial reluctance to come to therapy made the therapist question if she could form a meaningful bond with the child.

During supervision sessions, Pamir's therapist "marked the task" as reflecting on how she could help Pamir feel safe and at the same time allow him to incorporate difficult feelings into play without getting too disorganized. The therapist brought segments from her therapy sessions with Pamir during which he was immersed in his play in a way where there was a diffusion between his personal experience and the boundaries of play (e.g. suddenly starting to talk in first person narrative) and he was unresponsive to the therapist's interventions. The supervisor and the other therapists in the supervision group were curious about the therapist's feelings and how Pamir's play affected her. The therapist shared her feelings of being stuck, helpless, and not quite knowing how to be together with Pamir at these times. She couldn't understand his play and worried that her interventions wouldn't be effective, especially since Pamir was reluctant to come to therapy. As she shared these experiences, she realized that she was having a hard time mentalizing and remaining open to Pamir's communications. She felt detached, ineffective, and frustrated at times, while also blaming herself for having these feelings. The supervisory group then invited the therapist to imagine Pamir's experience during play. The therapist thought Pamir was also feeling quite helpless and unsafe, perhaps overwhelmed by difficult experiences he could not make sense of himself. The supervision group shared that they would feel similarly to the therapist, getting anxious and fearing not being able to help effectively. Thus, it was understandable that the therapist, under anxiety, might find herself in a non-mentalizing mode and struggle to remain curious and open. The therapist benefitted from having a place where she could reflect on her anxiety as the supervision group validated and shared her feelings and at the same time invited her to be curious about Pamir's feelings. The team afterwards invited the therapist to think about what Pamir may need at these times. The therapist and the supervisory group thought his need could be someone who can remain open to these difficult experiences, which were not fully formulated in their nature, validate their emotional intensity (just like the supervision group did for the therapist) and at the same time perhaps bring in elements of safety, such as "the safe shelter" metaphor when he got too dysregulated. In "returning to task", the therapist realized that her mentalizing capacity was influenced her confusion, forcing her to quickly understand Pamir and formulate what was going on, which was intensified further by the fear that he may drop out of therapy. This inhibited her capacity to remain "not knowing" and curious. With the help of the supervision group, she decided to remain open and at the same time occasionally intervene more actively to introduce elements of safety into Pamir's play narrative.

Initial phase of therapy (sessions 1–3)

The therapist started the first therapy session by introducing the calendar and the therapy box:

THERAPIST: I want to show you our therapy calendar. We are going to have 12 sessions together. Each square represents one session. For every session, you can draw something that reminds you of that session. We also have your therapy box here. I put down your name on it. We can keep the calendar inside and put everything we do together in the sessions. I'll always keep them here for you.

Pamir did not pay too much attention to the therapy calendar and the box. He wanted to start playing and instantly went to the sand tray. He took doll figures and placed them in the sand.

PAMIR: They are stuck inside the sand [referring to the figures he buried under]. They need to be rescued. Can you give me the police car?

THERAPIST: Oh, I remember we had played this last time. Yes, they were stuck last time as well. We were trying *so* hard to get them out. We can continue to save them. They really need our help. Dadi-dadi, the police are coming for help!

The therapist provided a narrative to the play, which seemed to have no beginning or ending in Pamir's mind. She brought in a context referencing the last time they played this. She then joined the play in pretend mode, using ostensive cues such as changes in her vocal tone to mark emotional states as pretend. This was crucial for Pamir, who, under the overwhelming nature of these emotions, could lose the as-if quality of play and experience the play themes as real.

PAMIR: They try to save them, but they are buried deep inside. They can't get out.

THERAPIST: Oh no! OK, let's keep trying. I wonder if we can approach from the other end of the sand.

PAMIR: The ambulance is coming, but there are people who are dead. There is too much sand [With a sudden shift in mood]. I don't want to play anymore. Let's close the sand tray.

THERAPIST: Ah, we tried very hard but it was difficult to try to continue saving them today. Perhaps, we can try another time, when we feel ready?

The themes expressed in play evoked acute anxiety in Pamir, diffusing the boundaries between pretend and reality. The therapist, understanding his need to distance himself from these emotions, remarked on the difficulty of the play theme and also suggested that this was something they could revisit when Pamir felt ready, giving him agency in play.

As Pamir started to explore the room, he found some toy darts and said with excitement, "Let's see who wins!" The therapist responded with enthusiasm, mirroring Pamir's excitement and slightly exaggerating it to mark the emergence of spontaneous affect. This was also an opportunity to acknowledge the child's intentional state of mind, which was to win, following a traumatic play theme that had left him feeling overwhelmed. At first, Pamir timidly threw the dart, but as the game progressed, he began to throw it harder. The therapist used attention control interventions, such as acknowledging and commenting on Pamir's behaviour, saying, "Wow, that was so fast!" or "Oh, now you are throwing harder". The aim of these interactions was to make Pamir aware of his body and different levels of force. This process was repeated many times during the early stages of therapy, helping Pamir to feel more at ease with his body and expressions.

In this phase of therapy, Pamir frequently went back to the themes of pain and hurt in his body. He said:

PAMIR: My tooth came out today. I pulled it out. It was hurting *so* much there.
THERAPIST: Oh, I see, it was hurting terribly.
PAMIR: Will all my teeth fall? Will my wisdom tooth fall as well? See, this one came out [showing the therapist the tooth that fell]. Will the ones at the very back come out again? Are they going to come out again?

Pamir had opened up his mouth widely, showing his teeth to the therapist and where it hurt. The therapist, at first, felt overwhelmed by the pressured nature of the questions. Then she thought to herself that Pamir was exploring a new way of being in his body, stronger, with more agency and intention. Then, these fears of losing his bodily intactness intruded. She did not make a remark about this. However, with a facial expression that showed much compassion towards the child's affect, she shifted her body to face Pamir, to communicate that she was ready to observe the pain he was showing, hold its intensity, and at the same time make him know that she was present, and they could think about this pain together. Pamir, in response to the openness and compassion of the therapist, which was again communicated via the use of ostensive cues, felt relieved. The forceful nature of the fearful questions diminished, and he could go back to playing.

During the initial phase, Pamir continued playing with rescue themes. However, gradually, his play narrative started to shift. It started to become more organized, with a more defined context, and he was able to introduce more protective characters.

PAMIR: This is a tank. These will be the soldiers. This is their commander. We have to *protect* the commander so he can protect the soldiers and help them prepare for war.

THERAPIST: Oh, I see. It is very important that we protect the commander so that he can protect the soldiers. Then, they can all feel safe to fight and defend themselves!

The therapist emphasized the importance of safety and protection; however, this time, she could do this within the play narrative the child had introduced without having to bring in the structure herself. Pamir started to prepare the soldiers for war, putting them next to each other one by one. He started to hum as he did this, clearly enjoying the play. In contrast to the prior play sequences, he seemed in charge of the play. Taking this opportunity, the therapist decided to stimulate the play narrative and encouraged Pamir to elaborate further on the different characters.

THERAPIST: Who are they fighting with?
PAMIR: The ones who want to conquer the world. The whites, reds, and blues are very powerful. Are there more soldiers there?

Pamir continued to play with the soldiers, imagining new scenarios and exploring different possibilities that led to mastery and growth. He then noticed the train and wanted to build a long railroad. He showed increased competence in mastering and manipulating the materials in the room. Eventually, Pamir incorporated the therapist into his symbolic play, expressing more agency.

PAMIR: Let's fight! You take this sword.

The therapist playfully joined the child, and they started fighting.

PAMIR: My sword is very sharp. Now let's also use guns.
THERAPIST: We have so many weapons to defend ourselves!

Middle phase (sessions 4–8)

The middle phase of therapy was marked by Pamir's growing awareness of himself and others. He started to be curious about the therapist and how she saw him. He arrived at one of these sessions late, and the therapist addressed this:

THERAPIST: You were a bit late today ... I have been waiting for you and wondering about you.

The therapist showed that she kept Pamir in mind, even when he was not there, bringing a sense of continuity to their meetings.

PAMIR: Yes, I've been working on my exams. We left home late. Are we going to have the same amount of time today?

THERAPIST: Ah, yes, we will end at the same time. But I wonder, when you asked, were you worried about having less time?

PAMIR: Does everyone have the same time? [looking sad] Do you play with other children here?

As Pamir developed ownership of the sessions, he began to express his worries about the fact that the therapy had a fixed end-point. Additionally, as his awareness of the other children in therapy grew, he became increasingly concerned about his place in the therapist's mind. The therapist thought that Pamir had not had an experience of being kept in mind as an individual with unique qualities that made him special among others. The therapist showed empathy and mentalized these concerns.

THERAPIST: You know Pamir, I was thinking about your questions. I wonder if you are concerned about our time together and whether it is unique to us.

Pamir nodded. The therapist also kept in mind the time-limited nature of MBT-C and took the opportunity to reintroduce the calendar. Previously, Pamir had merely made scribbles in the calendar and had not shown interest in filling it with more detail. The therapist thought that they could use the calendar as an opportunity to create their unique story.

THERAPIST: You remember our calendar? I have been thinking. It seems to me that it can help us see how we spend our time together, how much time we have left, and what has been unique to us in our sessions.

PAMIR: If I leave the calendar here I worry someone would throw it away.

THERAPIST: Pamir, I understand how worried you feel about safely expressing yourself. But no one can throw away your creations here. I always keep your box here safe, with your calendar inside.

As Pamir started to have the experience of being held safely in the therapist's mind and in the room, he said, "I know what I'm going to draw on my calendar this week. A drawing of myself and my cat." This was an important shift for him, marking a personal expression he felt secure enough to share.

Pamir's increasing awareness of how others viewed him also made him wonder if the therapist had kept him in mind and could notice changes in him:

PAMIR: Did you notice my hair? [He had been wearing a hoodie in the session until that moment but took it off.]

THERAPIST: Hmmm, let me see.

The therapist, at this point, made use of ostensive cues. She frowned, showing that she was thinking back to the last time, conjuring up an image of the child in her mind and comparing his facial features today, noticing differences.

THERAPIST: Oh, yes! Your hair was long last time and now it is short. You cut your hair!
PAMIR: My uncle cut it!

Pamir continued to make use of symbolic play during this phase of therapy. He wanted to play the story of a child. During the first sessions, he was also playing with children who needed to be rescued from the sand. However, in his initial sessions, the children had no name or identity. In his subsequent play, the child characters he chose were now inside the dollhouse and more clearly represented as individual people:

PAMIR: There is a child, who is 9 years old, and his sister. They are alone and their parents are dead.

The therapist made sure to let him know that she was listening and accompanying him during this personal narrative. She thoughtfully considered Pamir's history, taking into account the absence of his father and his mother's frequent psychological unavailability. She realized that this may have caused Pamir to experience their absence as a significant disruption in care. However, she decided not to draw any direct connections between the play themes and his real-life experiences. Instead, she assured him she was there with him throughout this painful story, and paid close attention to his emotional state. The play session provided a safe space for the child to narrate his story in a pretend mode.

PAMIR: The child has a sister who is looking after him. The child wakes up, now. The sister prepares food for them.

The therapist realized that the sister could have been her, but she did not make any direct links to the transference implications. Instead, she asked more about the sister and their relationship.

PAMIR: They play together. They have fun.

The therapist and Pamir continued to talk about "the child" and "the sister's" relationship through the metaphor of play. The therapist realized that the pretend world of play created a safe environment to process his own personal history. The play space provided the containment he needed to metabolize major life events. There was also a chance for revision as he brought in protective characters (e.g. the sister) that could attend to his needs. At the same time, gradually, Pamir started to share personal life events with the therapist.

PAMIR: Something happened recently. I want to tell you about that. I got a low grade from my exam and my mom got mad at me. We had a fight. My mom was really sad.

The safety of the therapy relationship allowed Pamir to reflect more on significant relationships in his life. There was also a clear improvement in his ability to mentalize his experiences. He could use mental state words such as "sad", make references to others' mental states, and link these to behaviours.

Review meeting

In this session, both therapists, the mother and Pamir reviewed the progress made so far. Pamir was now happy to attend therapy and he reported that his relationship with his mother had improved. He could express his anger in more constructive ways, defend his point of view, and resolve conflicts from his mother's perspective. The therapists and the family decided to prepare for the ending of therapy.

Final phase (sessions 10–12)

The final three sessions were an opportunity to process the upcoming ending and internalize the gains made in therapy. At the beginning of the first of these sessions, the therapist reminded Pamir that they had three sessions left. Pamir initially appeared unresponsive. However, soon he started complaining about pain in his body, mentioning that his head and eyes hurt. In response, the therapist showed empathy and asked him to describe the pain, its location, and how he felt it. Pamir explained that his eyes hurt a lot. The therapist thought to herself that the pain the child was experiencing could be due to the separation, a pain that he felt in his body but could not yet verbalize. She refrained from explicitly linking the pain to the separation since the physical sensations were too intense, limiting the child's capacity to mentalize. Nonetheless, the therapist took the bodily signals as a form of communication, both physical and mental pain. She continued to attend to the pain and inquired about its intensity, and Pamir responded that his eyes hurt only when he looked into the light. Then he mentioned that his finger hurt a lot, as he had hit it at school. The therapist expressed compassion and acknowledged the pain in her tone of voice and facial expression, saying, "There is so much hurt today, so much pain all over your body." Pamir then showed his ear, saying it was red and felt hot.

The therapist suggested that they both close their eyes and try to "feel" their body, in the form of a body scan. They started to focus their attention on different parts of the body, starting with the face, and then moving down to different parts. They paid particular attention to the parts of the body that hurt. The therapist asked how each part of his body felt, bringing in mental state language to enhance second-order representations of bodily states. Pamir started to become curious not only about how he felt inside but also about how the therapist felt. He started asking her how different parts of her body felt, which turned into a game where they both mentioned a body part and how it felt. By being able to explore physical sensations from within, Pamir felt more at ease which allowed his mentalizing to come back online. The therapist took the opportunity and suggested they now try to guess some aspect of each other's personality, something about what made them unique and what they could keep in mind about each other. However, Pamir closed his eyes and insisted that the therapist ask questions about him. Sensing that Pamir needed someone to be genuinely curious about his mind at that moment, she decided to played along:

PAMIR: OK! But you ask me something.
THERAPIST: OK, Pamir, what is your favourite food?
PAMIR: I like a special dish made out of beets.
THERAPIST: Ah, really? I have never heard of that dish before. I have learned something new about you.
PAMIR: Ask me another question!
THERAPIST: Pamir, what is your favourite subject at school?
PAMIR: Math, language, and social studies.
THERAPIST: Oh, wow! You have so many interests!

The therapist gently kept on asking questions about Pamir, which made him feel more engaged and interested in himself. He then shared his wish to get a pet fish and started talking about how he could feed it. The separation may have brought up fears of being forgotten. However, the therapist's careful attention to all aspects of Pamir during the session, including his physical sensations and mental attributes, provided a sense of security that he would be kept in mind.

In the following sessions, the therapist aimed to consolidate the narrative of their therapy. She went back to the focus formulation and the story of the sea shells:

THERAPIST: What do you think happened to the sea shells?

Pamir moved to the sand tray and took a toy shovel and hammer, then meticulously began to dig the sand in response to this question. The therapist recalled how they searched for the sea shells under the sand. Pamir continued to dig the sand, all the while hitting the surface with a hammer:

PAMIR: I am making the ground more solid and stronger! So the seashell don't sink in.
THERAPIST: Ahaa ... I see ... Initially, there was no safe ground on which the sea shells could stand. The sea shells are now firmer ground. They can stand there safely.

The therapist mentalized the child's play in metaphor, thinking that the solid ground may represent their therapy:

THERAPIST: It was quite a journey to find the sea shells and place them on solid ground during our therapy. I am remembering this entire journey...

The idea of remembering brought to Pamir's mind the desire to photograph himself playing in the room. In their final session, he brought his small camera and they took different pictures of the games they created in the room: one next to the sand tray, another enacting the sword game from the first sessions, another with the toy soldiers, and one next to the doll house. They matched these with the timeline they drew on the calendar. These pictures and the calendar gave them a solid way to remember the work that they had done together, to internalize meaningful aspects, and say goodbye.

Conclusion

In his early childhood, Pamir suffered from intense distress, disrupting his ability for mentalization and self-regulation. Mentalizing is a developmental achievement that primarily occurs within a secure parent–child relationship. When a child's emotional experiences and mental states are accurately responded to by the caregivers, the child starts to develop an understanding of their internal experience and a curiosity and openness towards mental states. However, in the context of early adversities, the child often misses out on such mentalizing experiences, and instead, their internal experiences are reflected back inaccurately and, at times, in a frightening way. Thus, the child may begin to avoid exploring others' minds as an adaptive response and/or develop mistrust in others' minds (i.e. epistemic mistrust). Pamir presumably developed in such a context. Finding a therapist who was curious about his mind and who understood his experiences helped relax his epistemic vigilance.

Although play is a fundamental part of MBT-C, Pamir was initially unable to engage in symbolic play. He struggled to complete his play narratives, which showed repetitive, traumatic themes. The distinction between reality and play often became blurred. The therapist helped Pamir differentiate what he felt inside and what was in the external world, via the use of ostensive cues such as responding with facial expressions that match and slightly exaggerate the child's internal states or changing her vocal tone to mark his emotional states. Eventually, with the help of the therapist's mentalizing of his play narrative, Pamir started to develop the capacity for symbolic play. The transitional play space gave Pamir many opportunities to metabolize major life events and play out new ways of being. He was able to discover a more agentful self and incorporate the themes of protection and defence he needed into his play. Throughout this process, the therapist ensured that the child felt safe in his explorations and affirmed his expressions. She maintained most of the communication in the play, so that he could process difficult emotions within the safety of the play relationship.

It is important to note the time-limited nature of MBT-C at this point. The therapist used the therapy box and calendar to actively work within the time limit, helping Pamir build his own therapy story and conclude therapy. Throughout the therapy, she aimed to keep the emerging themes in the here-and-now of the therapeutic relationship, to help the child regain the capacity to play, and modulate emotions. She made these without explicitly referring to the child's history. Due to the fragility of Pamir's capacity for mentalization and emotion tolerance, it was necessary to initially focus on developing the building blocks of mentalization such as joint attention and affect regulation before moving on to more explicit mentalization work. Towards the end of therapy, Pamir had a better capacity to mentalize his own experiences, more trust that he could be kept in mind by others, and regulate his emotions

As previously stated, Pamir's therapy took place within the context of a clinical trial (Halfon et al., 2024) conducted at IBUPC. The primary aim of the trial was to investigate the effectiveness of MBT-C compared to a parenting and child social skills group. Families completed specific scales assessing child symptoms, parent and child emotion regulation, parental mentalizing, and parenting stress at regular intervals during and after treatment to measure progress and assess its sustainability. The study results showed that children in the MBT-C group showed significantly greater reductions in their symptoms at the 6-month follow-up assessment compared to the control group. Additionally, both children and parents in the MBT-C group demonstrated significantly greater improvements in their ability to regulate emotions at the end of treatment, and these improvements were maintained at the follow-up assessment. Previous research conducted at IBUPC also showed that adherence to mentalizing principles in psychodynamic child psychotherapy improved children's affect regulation and symptoms (Halfon and Bulut, 2019).

When reviewing specific outcome results from the scales completed by Pamir and his mother, we observed substantial improvements in multiple areas. At the beginning of treatment, Pamir presented with clinical levels of externalizing and internalizing problems, along with significant emotion dysregulation. By the end of treatment, his problems had shifted to the non-clinical range, and there was a notable decrease in his emotional lability. Similarly, there was a major reduction in the mother's parenting stress. She also developed an interest and curiosity in her child's mind, along with improved mentalizing and emotion regulation. The improvements in Pamir's and his mother's functioning during therapy, as reported in the case study, along with the positive changes observed in the outcome scales, provide additional insight into the effectiveness of the therapeutic process.

Notes

1 The clinical trial was supported by the Scientific and Research Council of Turkey (TÜBİTAK) Project No: 121K733.
2 The patient and his parent were informed before the therapy process about research procedures. The mother provided written informed consent, and the child provided verbal assent concerning using their data, including questionnaires, videotapes, transcripts of sessions, and therapists' notes for research purposes. The case material has been de-identified to protect patient confidentiality. Patient names have been changed, and all identifying background information has been removed.

References

Bretherton, I., Prentiss, C., & Ridgeway, D. (1990). Family relationships as represented in a story-completion task at thirty-seven and fifty-four months of age. *New Directions for Child Development*, 1990 (48), 85–105. doi:10.1002/cd.23219904807.

Chazan, S., Kuchirko, Y., Beebe, B., & Sossin, K. M. (2016). A Longitudinal study of traumatic play activity using the children's developmental play instrument (CDPI). *Journal of Infant, Child, and Adolescent Psychotherapy*, 15 (1), 1–25. doi:10.1080/15289168.2015.1127729.

Halfon, S., Besiroglu, B., Bulut-Ozer, P., Aydın, G.İ., Epözdemir, Ş., Koç, H.B., Sözüer, B., Özsoy, Ö., Tulum, O., Tülü, S., & Midgley, N. (2024). The efficacy of mentalization-based treatment for children with internalizing and externalizing problems: A randomized controlled trial. *Journal of the American Academy of Child and Adolescent Psychotherapy*, online ahead of print. doi:10.1016/j.jaac.2024.12.006.

Halfon, S. & Bulut, P. (2019). Mentalization and the growth of symbolic play and affect regulation in psychodynamic therapy for children with behavioral problems. *Psychotherapy Research*, 29 (5), 666–678. doi:10.1080/10503307.2017.1393577.

Sunar, D. & Fişek, G. O. (2005). Contemporary Turkish families. In J. L. Roopnarine & U. P. Gielen (eds), *Families in global perspective* (169–183). Allyn & Bacon.

Target, M., Fonagy, P., & Shmueli-Goetz, Y. (2003). Attachment representations in school-age children: The development of the Child Attachment Interview (CAI). *Journal of Child Psychotherapy, 29(2)*, 171–186.

Chapter 7

Unravelling traumatic "luggage" and paving the way to mentalization-based treatment

The case of Yurko

Natasha Dobrova-Krol and Nicole Muller

It was there my mother gave me birth
And, singing as her child she nursed,
She passed her pain to me ...
Taras Shevchenko, 1846

Introduction

When working with children traumatized and displaced because of war, it's crucial to look beyond war-related circumstances. Such factors as economic deprivation, social hostility, isolation, and stressful life events have a significant impact on child development affecting openness to social learning, epistemic trust and mentalizing capacities (Luyten et al., 2020). A cultural-developmental approach to psychopathology seeks to integrate the role of the wider social and cultural environment, rather than being narrowly focused on the role of the immediate caregiving context or isolated traumatic event (Fonagy et al., 2022).

In this chapter we describe the preliminary phases of the mentalization-based treatment (MBT) at the National Psychotrauma Centre in the Netherlands of a Ukrainian boy and his family who had experienced trauma across multiple dimensions. Building on the time-limited model of MBT with school-age children (Midgley et al., 2017), we focus on restoring safety, connectedness, understanding the family's suffering and coping mechanisms, and recovering epistemic trust. This sets the foundation for enhancing the family's mentalizing capacities and addressing complex trauma from a cultural-developmental perspective (Fonagy et al., 2019; Hanene et al., 2018).

This approach is crucial given the broader context of trauma experienced by many displaced Ukrainian families. Indeed, with more than ten million forcibly displaced Ukrainian children and adults, the war in Ukraine has caused one of the fastest large-scale displacements of people since World War II (UNICEF, 2024). These families often carry not only the immediate experiences and losses from the war but also pre-existing mental health conditions. Ukrainian families often bear the burden of collective trauma,

DOI: 10.4324/9781032713441-11

including genocide and oppression. Political misuse of psychiatry during Soviet times and the general lack of mental health literacy within the population significantly contribute to a deep-seated mistrust in mental health and stigmatization of mental health conditions (Dobrova-Krol and van IJzendoorn, 2017; Van Voren, 2013; Quirke et al., 2021). In host countries, these individuals face post-migration stressors that further exacerbate the risk and onset of psychological disorders (Boettcher and Neuner, 2022). The severe conditions children have endured during and after the war starkly contrast with their developmental needs and their right to a safe environment. (Bürgin et al., 2022; Frounfelker et al., 2019). However, at a time when parental support is crucial, parents themselves are often grappling with shared and preexisting traumatic experiences. This inevitably affects family dynamics and, consequently, the mental health of children (Hyland et al., 2023; McElroy et al., 2023; Mooren et al., 2022).

Acknowledging these dynamics is indeed crucial in therapeutic work with families who have experienced displacement due to conflict. Individual and collective trauma, along with the prevailing social climate, can lead to epistemic vigilance or mistrust, which, while adaptive and may enhance survival in context of social hostility, results in powerlessness and this immediate threat must be carefully navigated especially during the initial stages of building therapeutic relationships (Campbell and Allison, 2022; Fonagy and Allison, 2023).

Case description: Yurko (8 years old) and his family

As with many other Ukrainian families, Yurko's family, which includes his mother Oksana, father Riad, and his 3-year-old sister Yarina, fled the country to escape the full scale envision of Russian troops which began in 2022. In the first days of the invasion, his family was exposed to heavy shelling and fighting, with bombs landing near their house, ruthlessly damaging their neighbourhood, so the family took the decision to leave the country. During their six-day journey, the family was exposed to brutal war images: weapons, soldiers at checkpoints, bodies, and body parts of deceased citizens. Upon their arrival in the Netherlands, the family received a 20-square-meter room in a shelter for forcibly displaced Ukrainian families. Both parents secured employment, Oksana as a part-time cleaner and Riad as a construction worker. Yurko was enrolled in a local school. However, adapting to school life posed a significant challenge for Yurko, his teachers, and his parents. He showed disruptive behaviour, volatility, and occasional aggression. Yurko refused to speak, was growling in class, and often hiding under the table.

The teachers attributed Yurko's behaviour to the effects of war trauma and recommended seeking assistance from a mental health specialist. Recognizing the importance of reestablishing epistemic trust and creating a safe environment we decided to engage not only with Yurko and his parents but also with the wider network around the family. Schools can be a very important partner in this process providing a supportive mentalizing environment that fosters trust and facilitates the child's overall adjustment and recovery as was the case for Yurko.

Making contact and overcoming epistemic mistrust

When meeting a family for the first time, using ostensive cues to establish a sense of "felt truth" is essential for overcoming mistrust and gaining a deeper understanding of the family's background and challenges. When this happens, it can facilitate a smoother and more effective therapeutic journey from the very beginning (Fonagy & Allison, 2014). The initial contact with Yurko occurred through a volunteer from the municipal shelter, who called to explain that Oksana and Yurko were unwilling to attend the first meeting due to feeling overwhelmed, confused, and also because they did not trust anyone. The volunteer continued at length, citing their Ukrainian background with the belief that "normal people do not go to psychologists or psychiatrists there". However, the fact that the therapist (the first author) was originally from Ukraine, and capable of conversing with Yurko and his mother in their native language, provided a glimmer of hope.

After several unsuccessful attempts, the first telephone conversation with Oksana finally took place. She sounded tense and wary but realizing she could speak in Ukrainian she agreed to talk. Oksana confirmed that things were not going well at school. When behavioural issues became unmanageable and threatened to disrupt the class, teachers would send a disappointed face emoji to Oksana, signalling that her son needed to be picked up promptly. Due to the language barrier, this became the only means to communicate the teachers' concerns. Oksana started to receive these emojis almost daily, fearing to pick up the phone and becoming more and more frustrated with her son. School days became a torment for Yurko and her, as she later shared with the therapist. We agreed to focus on school and how to help Yurko adjust there. Validating Oksana's concerns, sharing her narrative in her own language, and focusing on a practical goal identified by her, seemed to open the door a little wider: the first appointment could be scheduled.

Meeting with the child and the family

During the first face-to-face meeting, Oksana arrived with her son and the volunteer, who had initially contacted us. The father could not join us as he had to work. Yurko, a slim boy with dark brown hair and big eyes, appeared very shy, avoiding eye contact, and offering only brief, one-word answers. He frequently sought physical contact with his mother and sat next to her with his arms crossed, occasionally making growling sounds. As the volunteer began to discuss the difficulties Yurko faced at school, he silently got up and left the room. Oksana promptly brought him back, sternly reprimanding him for leaving.

To ease the tension, stop the non-mentalizing comments and explore mother's perception of Yurko further, the therapist asked what Yurko was good at, leading his mother to mention his talent for drawing and caring for his sister. This seemed to relax Yurko a little. While alone with the therapist Yurko chose to draw a picture of his family while responding to questions by nodding. He spoke softly, keeping his gaze down, and appeared to be sad. He could tell the therapist what he liked: "Silence, black, soup, drawing". He preferred to be with his father, as his mother often insisted on homework, and he disliked school. Yurko proudly presented his drawing to his mother and the volunteer when they returned.

During the second meeting, Yurko appeared livelier but remained hesitant to discuss difficult topics, expressing only feeling "a bit tired and a bit nice". Despite validation of his feelings, Yurko insisted on showing only positive emotions, maintaining avoidance and vigilance. The therapist wondered if there were any other feelings present besides tiredness. However, Yurko quickly interjected, stating, "I want to show only nice things". He sought every opportunity to act and interact with the therapist on his own terms. Explicit mentalizing about his feelings and thoughts or his situation was not yet possible, because of his profound lack of trust in another human being, or in this case the therapist.

Yurko presented as a physically restless boy who, once more familiar with the environment, seemed to manifest his tension or emotions through fidgeting, moving around, assuming peculiar postures while sitting, and often engaging in aggressive behaviour towards his sister. These behaviours suggested that Yurko struggled to manage his emotions and seek comfort appropriately. It appeared as if he had little control over this tension. It was precisely these movements that drew comments or reproaches from his mother. Whenever Yurko seemed hurt by his mother's remarks, he would cover his face with his hands and hide behind the chair.

Once Yurko was alone, he seemed to be a bit more focused and preferred engaging in activities. When presented with a game about emotions, Yurko displayed a good understanding, accurately identifying and naming most emotions. However, when asked to provide examples of situations when he experienced these feelings, he explained that they all stemmed from not getting what he wanted. This seemed to indicate potential emotional deprivation or neglect that he might have experienced in the past or present. He seemed to be very observant and accurate in interpreting his mother's negative emotions. He could discern her affect and link it to feelings of upset, disappointment, or anger. Indeed, studies suggest that children exposed to early negative relational experiences may develop a heightened sensitivity to negative emotions, which may be an adaptive response to their harsh environments (e.g. Pollak & Sinha, 2002). Considering factors like inter-generational trauma, attachment insecurity, and physical traumatic experiences compounded by the threat of war, it is not surprising that Yurko presented with a range of challenging behaviour. This included a preference for activities over verbal expression, difficulty articulating his own emotions, emotional regulation through avoidance, denial, splitting or aggression toward his sister, as well as acute observation of his mother's negative emotions. This range of behaviours suggested that he had experienced complex trauma and was showing an adaptive response to a harsh environment. In our assessment, we further focused on Yurko's attachment relationships and the impact of trauma on his emotional regulation and behaviour.

When choosing animals to represent his family, Yurko made choices that indicated the potential presence of some secure attachment representations alongside more potentially dangerous figures (for example his father as a shark). Although Yurko didn't use much language to express his internal world, he demonstrated that when given playful and safe space he could communicate about his relational experiences. This facilitated entry into more explicit mentalizing and engagement through symbolic play, enabling a deeper exploration of his emotions and relationships in the later stages of treatment.

In a subsequent session Yurko started to play more symbolically, choosing to show tanks and soldiers from both the Russian and Ukrainian armies engaged in intense combat. Subsequently, a character named Igor, depicted as a monster, entered his narrative, attacking the soldiers and trying to consume them. Yurko explained that Igor was enraged because the soldiers were trying to kill him and would not leave him alone. During the next session, Yurko chose guns and a helicopter, portraying them as attackers attempting to shoot and eliminate Yurko. The therapist could be with Yurko, present and containing, but not taking part in the play. It felt important and meaningful: Yurko seemed to be conveying a narrative about the world outside and inside him that was threatening and full of conflict.

Traumatic luggage

Although the recent war-related traumatic events seemed to be in the foreground, further assessment and exploration of Yurko's developmental history revealed that he had also been impacted by several traumatizing early circumstances, including both external and relational factors.

Yurko had a difficult start in life. His mother underwent a C-section due to the baby's asphyxia in utero. In the first six months following his birth, she experienced postpartum depression. Since birth, Yurko received medical treatment for his neurological condition. He exhibited restlessness, "his chin and legs were shaking, he was crying a lot, and slept very little", according to his mother. From the age of two he had become calmer. Yurko has also undergone several very painful medical and dental procedures, without anaesthesia. These experiences could have had a profound effect on his attachment and relational capacities, as well as his affective development and sense of self (Bowlby, 1980; Fonagy, 2018). Oksana believed that Yurko's current behaviour was primarily influenced by his experiences during the war. Yurko himself shared that he continued to recall frightening war images and avoided any war-related content shown on TV. He mentioned having difficulty falling asleep, frequent nightmares, and struggling to wake up early. Yurko slept with a night lamp on and always took his cuddly toy Huggy Wuggy to bed.

Yurko exhibited symptoms consistent with post-traumatic stress disorder. However, the observed negative interactions between him and his mother, as well as reported instances of harsh discipline by both parents, indicated the importance of addressing potential developmental trauma. This led us to work with him and his parents from an attachment and mentalization-based perspective.

Prolonging the pre-treatment phase and working on safety and epistemic trust

Conversations with Yurko's mother indicated that both parents were affected not only by the war and displacement stress but also by attachment and transgenerational trauma. Their difficulties in settling in the Netherlands, lack of privacy, conflicts in the refugee shelter, extreme worry for relatives and friends remaining in dangerous situations in Ukraine, and their own uncertain status all pointed to current chronic stress and the risk of re-traumatization (Boettcher & Neuner, 2022).

Identifying the focus for the work and starting treatment seemed indeed like "moving the furniture in a burning house". Individual symptoms of family members and the powerlessness of teachers at school, overwhelmed by Yurko's behavioural difficulties, continued to worsen the situation. Therefore, the primary focus at this stage was on establishing safety and finding meaning. We focused on fostering connectedness and trust and gradually unravelling the personal baggage of trauma within the family. We also tried to understand and recognize their coping mechanisms and strengths. This approach aimed to pave the way toward a shared understanding and treatment focus, realizing that we could only move forward if we established a positive relationship with Yurko and his mother. This would minimize the possibility of early drop-out, a common issue among forcibly displaced Ukrainian families.

Explaining confidentiality, especially regarding our interactions with third parties like the school, seemed to alleviate some of Oksana's concerns and bolster her feeling of being in control. When asked about how we could help and what tasks she would assign us, Oksana said, "Help my son. Teach him how to manage his emotions, listen to others, and develop trust in both others and his parents." At this point, Oksana did not feel it was necessary to address her relationship with Yurko, and we respected her position. However, Oksana told us that since the beginning of the war she felt tense and anxious most of the time, experienced intrusive traumatic memories, slept poorly, and suffered from frequent nightmares. Living in the shelter worsened her distress.

She engaged easily in verbal and physical conflicts with her neighbours, her husband, and her children. Oksana appeared to be at the end of her energy and mentalizing capacities. However, although introducing the theme of self-care resonated with Oksana, at this stage she was not yet ready to address her own mental well-being in therapy.

We agreed to hold weekly meetings with Oksana and Yurko. Additionally, we initiated contact with the school to enhance the basic level of safety and predictability in Yurko's environment and to ensure consistent support and engagement with Oksana by various means. Providing psychoeducation about trauma appeared to be beneficial for both Oksana and Yurko. The sense of guilt and responsibility previously imposed on Yurko for his "bad behaviour" began to transform into a comprehension of his behaviour as an "understandable reaction to abnormal circumstances". This shift in perspective created more room for the recovery of mentalization in both mother and child, allowing for greater insight and understanding into the parents' experiences and reactions.

We introduced MacLean's Triune Brain model using puppets, animal masks, and pictures. This playful approach represented the brain as an owl (for rational thinking), dolphin (for emotions and social connection), and crocodile (for survival instincts and fight-or-flight responses) (Siegel, 2024). It helped the family learn to recognize and communicate about different emotional states and their underlying reasons and needs within oneself and others and provided a vocabulary to communicate about them. This enabled the therapists to begin offering strategies for calming down and restoring mentalization. Oksana expressed interest in sharing these materials with Yurko's father Riad. However, getting Riad on board proved to be challenging. Riad, originally from Morocco, had lived in Ukraine for the past 15 years. Despite his migration, he preserved his family's and cultural traditions in his approach to parenting his children. According to Oksana, he was sceptical about the process and strongly believed in physical discipline and strict parenting approaches based on his own upbringing. Despite Oksana's own tendencies towards strictness and punitive measures in dealing with Yurko's behavioural issues, she expressed concerns about the potential harm of physical discipline.

While she was eager to involve the father, Oksana also worried about his reluctance to cooperate. After several unsuccessful attempts, the first telephone conversation with the father took place. During this conversation, we emphasized our recognition of his expertise and knowledge as a father and asked for his insights to better understand his son, with the goal of enhancing our effectiveness. Involving the father as an expert on his child seemed to open the door. He shared his observations, drawing parallels between Yurko's behaviour and his own childhood experiences. He also spoke warmly about Yurko and provided valuable insights into his son's character. Additionally, he agreed to meet with our male psychiatrist to discuss how we could further support Yurko. The decision to involve our male colleague was made with the intention of helping the father feel more at ease and open with another man.

The meeting with the psychiatrist, who not only conducted the psychiatric evaluation but also spoke "as a father to a father", proved to be reassuring, and introduced a sense of realistic hope. This meeting played an important role in establishing positive cooperation with both parents and addressing potential cultural sensitivities.

Working with school

With the parents' permission, we started to work with Yurko's two highly engaged but overwhelmed schoolteachers. We aimed to validate the teachers' efforts, provide psychoeducation about the impact of trauma on school performance, behaviour and development of the child, and share materials on trauma-sensitive education, to re-establish and strengthen their motivation to support Yurko effectively. We emphasized the concept of the "invisible luggage" (Horeweg, 2019) of trauma that Yurko carries, which contributed to his "double and even triple deprivation" that was impeding his development and making it a challenge for him to feel secure in new circumstances and to learn from others (Emanuel, 2002). This "invisible luggage" was also depriving him of the care and new restorative learning experience that he truly needed (Vliegen et al., 2023). Keeping in mind possible impact of the deprivation and invisible luggage on Yurko and its manifestation at school we agreed to focus on improving communication and implementing strategies such as "time out" or "recovery" moments at school with the help of the school psychologist who was assisting Yurko on a regular basis, helping to promote a sense of safety and predictability. Another aspect was focusing on reducing school-related stress at home. During one of the meetings, the teachers informed us that Yurko had shared information about the "crocodile, dolphin, and owl brain". Such integration of concepts from our sessions into the school environment contributed to fostering greater epistemic trust across settings.

While we were still working on establishing a shared understanding and treatment focus, with a primary emphasis on physical, emotional, and educational safety, a Dutch-speaking colleague started with play sessions with Yurko, the Ukrainian speaking therapist continued to work with the parents.

Play sessions with Yurko

In the weekly sessions with Yurko, our focus was on fostering predictable and continuous physical space and time in which he could feel included, seen, validated, and contained. This involved alternating between settings such as a playroom and gym, engaging in symbolic play and psychomotor activities, and allowing him to choose play materials and activities. We also incorporated elements of both following and leading in our interactions with Yurko, to ensure that he felt empowered and respected but also so that he learned to take turns and appreciate the safety of external boundaries.

Separation and reunion

The theme of separation and reunion was prominent throughout Yurko's therapy sessions. While Yurko typically engaged well with the child therapist and didn't hesitate to separate from his mother initially, he often sought his mother out during the sessions. Sometimes, this need for reunion seemed driven by separation anxiety, while at other times it was a search for validation, regulation, or a concern about his mother's well-being. During these brief reunions, Yurko would often inquire whether his mother had cried and for what reason. The topic of traumatic separation became more explicit towards the end of sessions when Yurko either resisted leaving the therapy room or engaged in conflicts with his mother. These instances possibly reflected Yurko's recent painful experiences of separation and loss connected with the war. These moments of separation made the therapist feel helpless amid the intense emotional reactions and unfolding affective storms. Maintaining a steady presence, validating emotions, and providing containment helped create a sense of safety and continuity in the therapeutic relationship. Reflecting on these feelings first with the co-therapist then a supervisor, and then in later sessions with the family, allowed for discussion of the painful moments of separation and loss, which helped the family begin to process these experiences.

Despite the dramatic nature of separations at the end of sessions, Oksana reported that Yurko was usually very quiet or asleep in the car on his way home. This suggested that potential reenactment and containment of dramatic separations during sessions helped to alleviate tension and anxiety, ultimately leading to a sense of calmness.

Working with "belligerence"

Exposure to war and violence, as well as harsh discipline, can deeply traumatize children, making their own aggressive impulses feel unsafe (e.g., Punmaki, 2002; Winnicott, 1986). Children who have experienced war-related trauma may resort to aggression as a means of coping with feelings of fear, helplessness, and loss, as well as a way of regaining control in a chaotic and threatening environment. Yurko consistently struggled with physical tension, restlessness, and aggressive outbursts both at school and at home.

Engaging in physical movement and play in the safe space of the gym, which Yurko preferred over the playroom, allowed him to release his physical tension. It also facilitated a deeper acquaintance with his physical sensations and experiences, allowing him to externalize in a safe environment his inner struggles and explore both the destructive and constructive aspects of anger and aggression, as well as learn about healthy boundaries. Through this process, he began to gain a sense of mastery over his overwhelming experiences.

Playing "tag" and "hide and seek"

For several sessions, Yurko consistently chose to play "tag" and "hide and seek". He would agitatedly run away or hide, often reversing roles and repeating these actions. Beyond the developmental themes such as separation and individuation, the search for connection and recognition, the repetitive, coercive and serious character of this play suggested they conveyed deeper traumatic meanings. Given Yurko's experiences of war, it seemed that he was reenacting these traumatic events. Observing that Yurko was not reacting and seemed to be in a closed system of self-regulation (Novick and Novick, 2016), the therapist recognized a need to contain and endure this lack of explicit contact. The therapist responded by continuing to offer a safe space, staying with him through difficult moments, and conveying the message that he was not alone. Discussing these challenges with a co-therapist and supervisor further informed her approach, ensuring that she could maintain the necessary containment within the therapeutic space.

Building a hut

During one of his play sessions, Yurko introduced a new element to his play routine by building a hut which seemed to symbolize his attempt to create a safe space or refuge. Perhaps it was also a representation of his fragile inner world in need of a safe shelter. After building the hut, Yurko often demolished it. In supervision sessions, we wondered whether the hut may also represent the shelter where the family had to stay during times of acute threat to their lives and providing a safe space for Yurko to take on the role of the aggressor. This may have allowed him to experience a sense of empowerment, contrasting to his feelings of helplessness and vulnerability and helping to restore his sense of control over these emotions.

During later sessions, the child therapist validated and contained Yurko's destructive urges through the calm presence, subtitling and providing safe space as he demolished the hut, staying focused in his aggression and seemingly finding some enjoyment in the act. Eventually, as his body tension subsided, Yurko chose to engage in quieter activities. This play repeated over several sessions. At the end of one such session, Yurko wrapped himself in a mat. When his mother came into the room as the session ended, he was lying in the foetal position, sucking his finger, possibly expressing his deep longing for safety and care.

The child therapist relied mostly on nonverbal interactions with Yurko, which appeared most appropriate at that stage. By staying attuned, seeking moments of joint attention, and simply being present with Yurko, the therapist mirrored him through gestures, facial expressions, and sounds, validating his individuality and strength at the same time as ensuring safe boundaries. This gentle connection facilitated the processing of the painful psychomotor content. Mentalizing in the team and with the supervisor further helped create a mentalizing context in the gym. This collaborative effort allowed the therapist to gain insights into Yurko's inner world and tailor interventions to meet his needs effectively, despite the language barrier.

Yurko's relationship with the therapists gradually evolved from merely engaging them as an audience to seeing them as facilitators who helped him understand and express his thoughts and feelings. He began to invite the therapist to play with him, such as hiding together during hide and seek, indicating a growing trust and comfort with their presence. Yurko also started to express enjoyment of his play sessions and even wished to prolong them. As the therapy progressed, Yurko displayed a caring side, particularly when the therapist returned after being ill. He took the initiative to engage in pretend play as a doctor, showing concern for her well-being by prescribing medicine for her cough. This showed his growing ability to express empathy and nurture a sense of connectedness.

An end-of-session ritual of playing together with his mother and both therapists that we introduced to model shared, positive experiences and playfulness as well as more healthy emotional exchange became a significant moment of reconnection for Yurko. During the last 10–15 minutes, the therapists encouraged Oksana to engage in play following Yurko's lead. They emphasized the importance of connecting through the pleasure of play. As Oksana began to enjoy these playful moments, they later discussed the positive experiences and their impact on their relationship. Even though this ritual was frequently disturbed by conflict, Yurko seemed to eagerly anticipate these moments of shared pleasure. This ritual likely served as a source of comfort and stability for Yurko amidst the challenges he faced, fostering a sense of safety, connection and belonging within the therapeutic environment. The presence of a supportive volunteer, who helped with transportation, further contributed to the sense of a safety network and trust for the family that helped to embrace the routine of the weekly sessions.

Moving small steps forward

Oksana reported that Yurko's father took the advice of the psychiatrist very seriously, and arranged quality father-son time, allowing more positive interaction and playfulness in their relationship. Within four months of work the angry outbursts at home reduced from about four to one per week. The school reported that although Yurko was still very reserved, he seemed to be more relaxed, engaged more often in group activities and showed less temper tantrums. Nevertheless, maintaining a positive therapeutic environment remained challenging. Efforts to provide psycho-educational information about developmental, relational needs and trauma that would be directly relevant and timely, as well as the validation of Oksana's emotions, only resulted in transient mentalizing that was easily disrupted by even minor deviations from what Oksana considered the "proper" behaviour she expected from Yurko. A sense of chaos, overpowering emotions, and non-mentalizing interactions from Oksana towards Yurko, including rejecting and humiliating reactions, still dominated their interactions with each other.

During one of the sessions, which began cheerfully and relaxed, the family brought a balloon to complete a school assignment – they had to photograph a balloon in a place where Yurko felt good. Fortunately, our centre was one of those places. The mood remained positive until the moment when Yurko failed to make the facial expression for the photo that Oksana had in mind. She became increasingly frustrated, accusing Yurko of not cooperating and being obstructive, and threatened to leave. Yurko initially covered his face with his hands and then crawled behind the chair. When the therapist took the lead and tried to intervene by sharing her understanding of the situation and validating the feelings of both Yurko and Oksana, Yurko resumed playing. However, it took more effort for Oksana to calm down.

Once Yurko left the room with the child therapist, Oksana commented: "You just need to give him a rabbit punch, then he quickly learns how to behave with other people". Although these words evoked deep concern for the safety of the boy and a strong desire to act and protect the child, we also tried to reflect on the tension and rage that Oksana constantly felt. She shared that she could not relax, haunted by painful memories and current news about the war. She was infuriated by problems and fights with fellow residents in the shelter. Containing and validating these feelings helped Oksana to calm down and to reflect on her own behaviour, acknowledging that she regularly lashed out at Yurko as if he was her punching bag. This became an important turning point when Oksana recognized her own need for support and treatment. We agreed that from now on, we would have separate sessions with Oksana about trauma and parenting and would explore individual treatment possibilities for her.

We referred Oksana to the team in the same clinic that worked with traumatized adults, hoping that this would help address her psychological suffering and disentangle her parenting from unresolved relational dynamics and painful experiences from her own history. We learned about multiple traumatic experiences that Yurko's mother faced in her own childhood. This helped us to recognize more vulnerable spots that could have been triggered in interactions with her son, reactivating "old sores" from her own history. The voices of the past, left by her childhood trauma, could have intruded into her present relationship with Yurko, impeding her ability to mentalize about emotionally painful experiences of fear and helplessness. This made Oksana vulnerable to identifying with the aggressor from the past rather than responding to the distress of the child in the here and now (Fraiberg et al., 1975; Fonagy, 1993). It seemed that Yurko's "unacceptable behaviour" triggered trauma-related ideation each time, creating an unmentalized alien core (Fonagy et al., 2002) around the child's experience and impacting Oksana's mirroring response. We wondered whether the alien parts of Oksana were projected onto the child, planting a seed for the development of the "alien self" in Yurko (Ensink et al., 2014; Novick & Novick, 2005). On another level, we assumed that the language of restraint, coercive discipline, and rebuke might also serve as her way of relating to her children – her "language of love and protection" – her utmost effort to promptly stop or eradicate the child's disturbing behaviour and ensure that Yurko would not turn out to be like her own father or grandfather who was a violent alcoholic.

For Oksana thinking together with the therapist about the possible meaning of Yurko's underlying behaviour remained challenging. At the same time, psychoeducation on trauma triggers in parenting and mirroring as the key to the development of identity, affective states, and self-regulation in a child seemed to evoke genuine curiosity, supporting her desire to learn and be a good parent (Novick & Novick, 2005). Oksana also actively shared her discoveries with her husband. Besides the harsh moments in Oksana's responses, there were also regular instances of warm and affectionate interactions when Yurko sought and received warm, reassuring hugs from his mother, even moments after the tumult of disciplinary measures. We began actively seeking opportunities to create more positive moments between Oksana and Yurko by encouraging the reassuring physical contacts between them. Gradually we introduced interventions aimed at slowing down Oksana's automatic reactions, providing her with the opportunity to delay her responses, and giving Yurko the space to express what was bothering or upsetting him. Gradually Oksana started to adopt a gentler approach towards her son. During one of the later sessions, when Yurko initially ran away from her but later returned and timidly peeked through the door, instead of her usual reprimand, Oksana approached him with tenderness. She softly inquired, "Are you OK? Would you like a kiss? Come, sit on my lap, and tell me." Yurko responded by approaching his mother, sitting on her lap, resting his head on her shoulder, and telling her why he ran away.

The therapist's own mentalizing process

For the first author, having a similar cultural background and history as the family, speaking the same language, and sharing anger, helplessness, and pain in the face of the atrocities of war seemed to facilitate the "moments of meeting" and mutual recognition (Benjamin, 1990; Campbell & Allison, 2022). On the other hand, the gradual unfolding of the layers of complexity and needs of Yurko and his family against the background of chronic stress and psychological suffering evoked counter-transferential feelings of overidentifying with Oksana's suffering and the temptation to collude with Oksana's representation of the outside world as overpowering. The therapist had to contain the feeling of urgency while also experiencing frustration with the constraints of the mental health care system and waiting lists, fuelled by "survivor guilt" and concern about the safety and emotional well-being of the child.

To manage and contain these counter-transferential reactions, the therapist established close cooperation with the child therapist. Before and after each session, they had a fine-tuning contact to check in with and update each other, to agree on the focus and possible interventions, or to reflect on the process and the content of the next session. This collaboration was supported by regular discussions within the team, as well as in external supervision groups and supervisions from the second author. All these measures helped the therapists to maintain and regain their mentalizing and to stay patient, hopeful, and appreciative of the small steps taken, understanding that the trust of the family had to be earned before further assistance could be accepted in their journey towards healing.

Moving on

This is an ongoing case where slow but significant progress is being made. By emphasizing these moments of connectedness, understanding, shared plea-sure, and playfulness, we aim to continue to encourage building on such interactions in the therapy room and at home and facilitate greater security in the attachment relationships between Oksana and Yurko. In this still unfold-ing therapeutic journey, and now that Oksana is also engaged in her own therapy, we are striving to involve Yurko's father in parenting sessions to build a cohesive narrative within the MBT framework. This approach aims to create a united parental strategy for addressing Yurko's emotional and psy-chological needs. By preparing the parents and strengthening family bonds, we hope they will be able to provide safety and assist Yurko in processing his traumatic memories. This collaborative effort focuses on building Yurko's narrative, ensuring he feels supported and understood by both parents.

Conclusion

The case of Yurko's treatment highlights several critical adjustments of the MBT protocol that were needed, in the context of the traumatic context, to enhance the effectiveness of the intervention and to create a more supportive and effective therapeutic environment. This included addressing both the visible and invisible complexities of developmental trauma in a context of war and migration:

1   **Prioritizing safety and stability**: Emphasizing safety, stability, consistency, and predictability was paramount, particularly in the initial stages of treatment. This phase, as Vliegen et al. (2023) suggest, is akin to prior-itizing "the glass over the wine", helped to foster relatedness and address epistemic mistrust.
2   **Extended initial assessment phase**: A thorough and extended initial assess-ment phase allowed a more comprehensive trauma symptoms and trauma

history assessment, of both child and parents, while considering broader transgenerational, socio-economic and cultural contexts. This phase also served to further establish and recover epistemic trust and recognize and address the "invisible luggage", contain the initial chaos or rather the complexity of the hidden burdens.

3   **Enhanced psychoeducation**: Providing extensive psychoeducation on the impact of complex trauma on development, emotions, and behaviour was vital for both children and their caregivers. It was necessary to revisit these topics repeatedly to ensure understanding and integration, helping both children and caregivers make sense of their experiences and reactions.

4   **Attention to the traumatization of parents**: In addition to MBT-Parent work, it was important to offer parallel treatment for parents themselves. Parents' unresolved trauma can contribute to an unsafe environment and retraumatization of children. Addressing their trauma is crucial for creating a more secure and supportive family dynamic. In MBT work with parents alongside the trajectory of the child, the focus was on acknowledging the impact of their trauma on the parental skills and on the relationship between parent and child in the past and present.

5   **Multidisciplinary collaboration**: Acknowledging the potential for secondary traumatization or over-identification by the therapist has been especially important. It required openness about the therapist's experiences and support from their team to recover and maintain mentalization. Engaging in extensive collaboration with other services and schools provided a more comprehensive support network for the family, thereby supporting the treatment process.

References

Benjamin, J. (1990). An outline of intersubjectivity: The development of recognition. *Psychoanalytic Psychology*, 7 (1), 33–46.

Boettcher, V. S. & Neuner, F. (2022). The impact of an insecure asylum status on the mental health of adult refugees in Germany. *Clinical Psychology in Europe*, 4 (1), article e6587.

Bowlby, J. (1980). *Attachment and loss, vol. 3: Sadness and depression*. Basic Books.

Bürgin, D., Anagnostopoulos, D., Vitiello, B., Sukale, T., Schmid, M., & Fegert, J. M. (2022). Impact of war and forced displacement on children's mental health: Multilevel, needs-oriented, and trauma-informed approaches. *European Child and Adolescent Psychiatry*, 31 (6), 845–853.

Campbell, C. & Allison, E. (2022). Mentalizing the modern world. *Psychoanalytic Psychotherapy*, 36 (3), 206–217.

Dobrova-Krol, N. & van IJzendoorn, M. (2017). Institutional care in Ukraine: Historical underpinnings and developmental consequences. In A. Rus, S. Parris, & E. Stativa (eds), *Child maltreatment in residential care*. Springer.

Emanuel, L. (2002). Deprivation × 3. *Journal of Child Psychotherapy*, 28, 163–179. doi:10.1080/00754170210143771.

Ensink, K., Berthelot, N., Bernazzani, O., Normandin, L., & Fonagy, P. (2014). Another step closer to measuring the ghosts in the nursery: Preliminary validation of the Trauma Reflective Functioning Scale. *Frontiers in Psychology*, 5, 1471.

Fonagy, P. (1993). Psychoanalytic and empirical approaches to developmental psychopathology: Can they be usefully integrated? *Journal of the Royal Society of Medicine*, 86 (10), 577–581.

Fonagy, P. (2018). Attachment, trauma, and psychoanalysis: Where psychoanalysis meets neuroscience. In J. Grotstein (ed.), *Early development and its disturbances* (pp. 53–75). Routledge.

Fonagy, P. & Allison, E. (2014). The role of mentalizing and epistemic trust in the therapeutic relationship. *Psychotherapy*, 51 (3), 372–380. doi:10.1037/a0036505.

Fonagy, P., Luyten, P., Allison, E., & Campbell, C. (2019). Mentalizing, epistemic trust, and the phenomenology of psychotherapy. *Psychopathology*, 52 (2), 94–103.

Fonagy, P., Campbell, C., Constantinou, M., Higgitt, A., Allison, E., & Luyten, P. (2022). Culture and psychopathology: An attempt at reconsidering the role of social learning, *Development and Psychopathology*, 34, 1205–1220 doi:10.1017/S0954579421000092.

Fonagy, P., Gergely, G., Jurist, E. L., & Target, M. (2002). *Affect regulation, mentalization, and the development of the self*. Other Press.

Fonagy, P. & Allison, E. (2023). Beyond mentalizing: Epistemic trust and the transmission of culture. *The Psychoanalytic Quarterly*, 92 (4), 599–640.

Fraiberg, S., Adelson, E., & Shapiro, V. (1975). Ghosts in the nursery: A psychoanalytic approach to the problems of impaired infant-mother relationships. *Journal of the American Academy of Child Psychiatry*, 14 (3), 387–421. doi:10.1016/s0002-7138(09)61442-4.

Frounfelker, R., *et al.* (2019). Living through war: Mental health of children and youth in conflict-affected areas. https://international-review.icrc.org/articles/living-through-war-mental-health-children-and-youth-conflict-affected-areas.

Hanene, L., Hannele, F., & Marja, T. (2018). Stories of trauma in family therapy with refugees: Supporting safe relational spaces of narration and silence. *Journal of Marital and Family Therapy*, 44 (3), 483–497.

Hyland, P., Vallières, F., Shevlin, M., Karatzias, T., Ben-Ezra, M., McElroy, E., Vang, M. L., Lorberg, B., & Martsenkovskyi, D. (2023). Psychological consequences of war in Ukraine: Assessing changes in mental health among Ukrainian parents. *Psychological Medicine*, 53 (15), 7466–7468.

Horeweg, A. (2019). Schoolbrede aandacht voor het getraumatiseerde kind. *Vakblad Beter Begeleiden*, 2019, 40–43.

Luyten, P., Campbell, C., Allison, E., & Fónagy, P. (2020). The mentalizing approach to psychopathology: State of the art and future directions. *Annual Review of Clinical Psychologe*, 16, 297–325.

McElroy, E., *et al.* (2023). Change in child mental health during the Ukraine war: Evidence from a large sample of parents. *European Child and Adolescent Psychiatry*, 33 (5), 1–8.

Midgley, N., Ensink, K., Lindqvist, K., Malberg, N., & Muller, N. (2017). *Mentalization-based treatment for children: A time-limited approach*. American Psychological Association.

Mooren, G.T.M., Bala, J., de Kok, M., Baars, J., & van Essen, J. (2022). *Handboek familierelaties bij psychotrauma: Diagnostiek en behandeling van kinderen en gezinnen*. Uitgeverij Boom.

Novick, K. K. & Novick, J. (2005). *Working with parents makes therapy work.* Jason Aronson Publishers.

Novick, J. & Novick, K. K. (2016). *Freedom to choose: Two systems of self-regulation.* International Psychoanalytic Books.

Pollak, S. D. & Sinha, P. (2002). Effects of early experience on children's recognition of facial displays of emotion. *Developmental Psychology,* 38 (5), 784–791.

Punamäki, R. L. (2002). The uninvited guest of war enters childhood: Developmental and personality aspects of war and military violence. *Traumatology,* 8 (3), 181–204. doi:10.1080/00207590244000133.

Siegel, D. J. (2024). Minding the brain: Dr. Daniel Siegel's hand model of the brain. www.psychalive.org/daniel-siegel-hand-model-brain/.

Shevchenko, T. (1846). If you but knew, trans. J. Weir. https://shevchenko.ca/taras-shevchenko/poem.cfm?poem=48.

Quirke, E., Klymchuk, V., Suvalo, O., Bakolis, I., & Thornicroft, G. (2021). Mental health stigma in Ukraine: Cross-sectional survey. *Global Mental Health,* 8, article e11.

UNICEF. (2022). More than half of Ukraine's children displaced after one month of war. www.unicef.org/press-releases/more-half-ukraines-children-displaced-after-one-month-war.

Van Voren, R. (2013). Psychiatry as a tool for coercion in post-Soviet countries. In D. Bhugra & S. Bhui (eds), *Textbook of cultural psychiatry* (pp. 313–328). Cambridge University Press.

Vliegen, N., Tang, E., Midgley, N., Luyten, P., & Fonagy, P. (2023). *Therapeutic work for children with complex trauma: A three-track psychodynamic approach.* Routledge.

Winnicott, D. W. (1986). Home is where we start from. In C. Winnicott, R. Shepherd, & M. Davis (eds), *Home is where we start from: Essays by a psychoanalyst* (pp. 112–120). W. W. Norton.

Chapter 8

Working with children in groups

Maria Højer Nannestad

Introduction

In Denmark, one in three children experiences their parents' divorce, and about one in six of these children encounter high levels of parental conflict, often involving custody disputes (Steinvig, 2022). Children's rights are highly prioritized in the Danish legal and social systems. However, an increasing number of parents use the courts and social services as part of their conflict, submitting repeated inquiries to authorities. Each time, social law mandates that children are listened to, resulting in children having to attend numerous meetings. Despite the well-meaning intentions of professionals who want to listen, many children feel caught in the system and feel that, by sharing their perspectives, they are forced to choose between their parents. This often feels overwhelming and like an immense responsibility for the children. Moreover, living with family violence inflicts severe trauma, impacting children's ability to form secure attachments and build trust.

This chapter describes a mentalization-based group treatment for children, with a focus on supporting those who have experienced trauma. It will highlight some key principles, including foundational approaches and specific interventions that can enhance mentalization and epistemic trust within the group. The clinical examples are drawn from a slow-opening group[1] of children aged 9 to 16 who have experienced trauma in the form of domestic violence. All children in the group have spent significant effort focusing on the violent parent and are often highly attuned to the well-being of the non-violent parent. They are accustomed to adjusting their behaviour in an attempt to manage the violence, frequently at the expense of attending to their own needs and inner lives (Graham-Bermann & Levendosky, 2011; Lieberman et al., 2015). The main focus in the group, which is run jointly by two therapists, is to support the children in mentalizing, processing their trauma, and addressing trauma symptoms. This is achieved by shifting the balance of attention from others to themselves, fostering epistemic trust, and building shared experiences of "we-ness". Collaboration with parents is crucial and can take various forms. Ideally, this includes a parallel mentalizing group for

DOI: 10.4324/9781032713441-12

parents, sometimes with joint sessions or multi-family therapy (Asen & Scholz, 2010). At a minimum, parents are involved in the initial assessment and final sessions to stay informed about the group's topics and support their child's development. Parents are encouraged to give their children permission to speak about traumas and any family taboos.

Introducing two group members: Ingrid (10 years old) and Amir (12 years old)

Ingrid joined the group when she was nine years old. She was born in a shelter due to physical and psychological violence from her father toward her mother and older sister. Although they moved away from the violence, it continued throughout Ingrid's childhood. She often overheard her parents arguing on the phone, and on several occasions, her father refused to return the children after weekend visits. Ingrid grew up with frequent meetings involving family court and social workers, as her father repeatedly sent letters to social services, claiming the children were being mistreated in their mother's care. Ingrid's mother, deeply affected by psychological stress, appeared sad and depressed, often spending much of her day on the couch and struggling to be emotionally available for Ingrid and her sister. Ingrid appears as a sad and worried child, concerned for her mother's well-being, though she loves her mother deeply and has many good memories with her and her sister. She is also frustrated with ongoing meetings with social workers regarding school absences, as well as with psychiatric services due to her own self-harm and depression. Ingrid feels that many people are trying to "fix" her, but she resists this. She once said, "In mental health services, they want me to go from A to B. In this group, I can be A, B, C, D, or E, and everything is OK. And in a weird way, that's what makes it possible for me to grow."

Ingrid attends the group because her mother spoke positively about a women's group she had attended. When she joined, Ingrid told us she did not trust psychologists, but she was motivated by the chance to meet other children who might understand her experiences. Ingrid's goal in the group is to work toward sharing some of the thoughts and feelings she has otherwise avoided, as she has only ever discussed her experiences of violence with her mother. In Table 8.1 Ingrid's mentalizing abilities are summarized.

Amir joined the group shortly after he and his family had returned home from a domestic violence shelter, where he had stayed with his mother, two older brothers, and younger twin sisters. Amir is a quiet, observant boy who enjoys playing piano, loves to read, and has a thoughtful perspective on the world. He also carries deep concerns for his family. Growing up, Amir and his siblings saw their father as "two-faced". On one hand, their father had a charming, cheerful side – he was social, talkative, well liked in their community, and many of Amir's friends even thought he was lucky to have such a friendly dad. However, their father also had another side, struggling with

Table 8.1 Ingrid's building blocks of mentalizing as she started the group.

Attention regulation	Ingrid sometimes drifts off with a sad expression and occasionally reaches for her phone as a distraction. It seems that inner struggles and past memories affect her ability to fully engage in the present moment.
Affect regulation	Ingrid presents as over-regulated on the outside, yet under-regulated on the inside. She often appears very calm, sometimes almost passive, but when she opens up about her emotional state, it becomes clear that she can feel deeply overwhelmed by her emotions.
Explicit mentalizing	Ingrid is often preoccupied with others and has complex theories about their mental states, typically viewing adults at school and in the psychiatric unit with a negative bias.
Focus	Building epistemic trust and supporting Ingrid in expressing and sharing her thoughts and feelings with the group at a pace that feels safe for her. Helping Ingrid develop self-awareness and offering her opportunities, through playfulness and positive experiences, to engage with the group.

anger management and capable of intense aggression. To some extent, Amir and his siblings learned to anticipate certain triggers for his father's anger, such as when they were noisy or fighting. Yet, at other times, their father's aggression felt completely unpredictable, leaving Amir confused and fearful. The violence took many forms. Amir recalls how his father would often pick him up, carry him into his room, and throw him forcefully onto the floor while yelling that Amir was a terrible child. He saw his older brothers endure the same treatment; they would scream and cry loudly, only for sudden silence to follow, which filled Amir with dread, fearing his father had hurt them fatally.

Violence had been part of Amir's life for as long as he could remember. One day, however, it escalated. He recalls walking into the kitchen to see his father holding a knife to his mother's neck. Amir froze, afraid any sound might provoke his father to act. Fortunately, a neighbour witnessed the incident, intervened, and called the police. This event led Amir, his mother, and his siblings to seek shelter. It took months in the group before Amir could share this experience, just as it took time for him to express his overwhelming fear of becoming violent like his father. Amir worried he might have a "monster" inside him that could one day awaken. He struggled with anxiety, sleep difficulties, self-criticism, and intense shame. Amir's goal in the group was to share the difficult thoughts and experiences that had haunted him, which he had never shared with anyone. Initially anxious about joining, Amir later described the relief of meeting other children who had faced similar experiences. For the first time, he felt truly understood.

In Table 8.2 Amir's mentalizing capacity is described. During the assessment phase, the therapist assesses the developmental level of a child to determine which building block of mentalization can be best targeted.

Table 8.2 Amir's building blocks of mentalizing as he started the group.

Attention regulation	Amir appears very present in the group, but his body can sometimes seem restless (e.g. we notice him tapping his feet), and he has small tics in his face and neck. Amir has to do a lot of schoolwork after class because he struggles to maintain focus during school hours. The teachers don't seem to notice this, and we wonder if we're able to pick up on all his signals within the group.
Affect regulation	Amir appears over-regulated on the outside, but we know that he can become overwhelmed by difficult emotions. He is very afraid of crying, fearing that he will fall apart if he does. When Amir discusses challenging topics, such as the fear of becoming violent like his father, his entire body reacts. He becomes very restless and seems to struggle to remain in the room.
Explicit mentalizing	Amir has advanced mentalizing skills for his age, but these abilities break down when his emotional arousal increases. He is more skilled at mentalizing others than himself and can be very harsh on himself, almost to the point of being punitive.
Focus	Supporting Amir in transferring his positive qualities of mentalizing others to also mentalizing himself. Helping him share and process some of his specific traumatic memories, both in group and individual sessions. When he contributes to the group discussion, our focus is on mentalizing and understanding his responses, both in the context of the situation and in the present moment.

The main principles of mentalization-based trauma treatment in group therapy with children

The explicit focus on mentalization, along with a careful, consistent application of core elements from the mentalizing model, defines this treatment approach. The principles of mentalization-based therapy for children and manuals for MBT groups for adults and adolescents have been combined to create a framework that allows children to benefit from mentalizing their trauma within a group of peers (Midgley et al., 2017; Muller & Dwyer-Hall 2021; Karterud, 2015).

Being in a group allows children to experience themselves in relation to others – not only peers of the same age but also those who are younger or older. As they listen to one another, the children's ability to mentalize is naturally activated. They shift between understanding others' perspectives and their own. For instance, when Ingrid and Amir joined the group, a 15-year-old girl named Fatima was already sharing her thoughts and feelings about vulnerable experiences from her life. Both Ingrid and Amir seemed to admire her and listened intently, with open minds. Fatima became a respected member of the group, providing a model for Ingrid and Amir to imagine themselves in the future. Likewise, as Fatima listened to Ingrid and Amir, she was able to reflect on her younger self through their perspectives. This group setting provides children with the chance not only to observe and respond to one another but also to be seen, heard, and valued by their peers and therapists. The group atmosphere helps children borrow language from each other, expanding their vocabulary and enabling them to articulate their own feelings. Hearing another child describe a familiar emotion they couldn't previously name allows children to respond, "I know that feeling", or "That could almost be me, except I …" – a liberating and validating experience. The group setting also lets children experience themselves as helpful and valued, reinforcing positive feelings that can carry into other relationships.

As group therapists, we find it deeply rewarding to witness moments of enhanced epistemic trust and "we-ness" among the children. When children succeed in mentalizing with each other's support, they experience an immediate sense of shared connection – a "we-mode" that stands in stark contrast to the isolation they felt due to trauma. These moments of connection significantly aid children in mentalizing their trauma. Amir once said, "I realize now that the other children weren't the cause of the violence in their families, and that makes me wonder if maybe I'm not to blame either." Building epistemic trust can take time, especially with long-term developmental trauma, but repeated experiences of "we-ness" play a crucial role in addressing the feeling of isolation that comes from surviving difficult and threatening situations (Vliegen et al., 2023).

When Amir finally felt safe enough to share his experience of fearing his father might kill his mother, he witnessed how his story created a serious yet compassionate atmosphere. Other children, who had felt similarly fearful for their family members' safety, understood him deeply. The words and expressions of the children and therapists helped Amir feel seen and understood. When a therapist asked how he felt after sharing and hearing others' responses, Amir replied, "I feel less alone, and like I could cry without falling apart." Later, he expressed pride in reaching a point where he could share this memory, previously burdened with isolation and fear. He was pleased when other group members told him that his courage inspired them to open up about their own traumatic memories.

The therapeutic stance and core principles

As with other forms of MBT, success in this treatment approach relies less on specific techniques and more on the therapist's stance and approach. The mentalizing stance emphasizes that therapists must be genuinely warm, empathic, engaged, non-judgmental, and deeply curious about all the children in the group (Midgley et al., 2017).

Children with traumatic relational experiences are often highly sensitive to others' mental states, as they have often been met in non-mentalizing ways and have witnessed loved ones treated in similar ways. For these children to feel safe enough to share their vulnerabilities, it is essential that they see their peers being treated with respect and understanding (Graham-Bermann &

Levendosky, 2011; Lieberman et al., 2015). Regulating arousal levels is key when mentalizing. Traumatized children may either experience sudden increases in arousal or be "skilled" at concealing their feelings, especially when arousal rises (Vliegen et al., 2023; Graham-Bermann & Levendosky, 2011). High arousal can lead to mentalizing breakdowns, which can quickly spread within the group. Group therapists play a crucial role in supporting both down- and up-regulation of arousal, shifting between serious topics and more neutral or light-hearted ones to sustain contact with mental states. Therapists may also encourage children to share their thoughts and feelings as a way to help a peer regain mentalizing abilities when slipping into "pretend mode".

A primary focus in group-based MBT is on mental states, interpersonal experiences, and helping children understand the impact of emotions, which is explained to children and parents before the group begins. This is especially vital for children with developmental trauma, as they may have limited awareness of emotional states and a tendency to interpret others' emotions negatively (Karterud, 2015). Thus, encouraging curiosity and exploration of emotions – both through reflection and play – is central to the approach (Midgley et al., 2017). Emotions that arise during sessions are emphasized and explored to help children recognize and respond to them in a meaningful way, something they often do naturally.

In our group therapy, we use an activity that fosters emotional exploration of interpersonal events. One child briefly describes an event without revealing their emotional state, and the group then guesses what thoughts or emotions might be involved. Ingrid once shared an incident where a teacher yelled at her and a friend, which a therapist sketched on the whiteboard. As the group explored Ingrid's experience, they speculated on different emotions, while the therapist recorded responses on the board. Both therapists contributed guesses to ensure a range of perspectives. In the end, Ingrid shared her feelings about the event and reflected on any new perspectives she gained from the group. The therapists then asked the children how they felt about the activity, here and now. Amir's situation presented a more sensitive dilemma: he had chosen not to see his father because of his father's violence, leaving his younger siblings to see him alone. The therapists checked with Amir and the group about exploring this event, and they agreed. This time, the group's tone became more thoughtful and serious. Afterwards, the children shared that they noticed feeling more sombre yet empowered by engaging with such meaningful topics.

Balancing attention among group members is essential, though it doesn't mean each child receives exactly equal focus. To keep children engaged and attuned, the therapist ensures a steady pace and alternates between active and passive participation. Though individual needs vary, it remains a key task for therapists to maintain this balance and keep each child in mind throughout the session.

Discussing group norms and fostering shared ownership of the group is essential. The therapist is responsible for setting boundaries and establishing group rules, but children actively participate in defining group norms and traditions. For instance, they discuss how to welcome new members or handle farewells. This involvement promotes a sense of coherence and agency – especially critical for children with developmental trauma, who may feel passive in their own lives (Lieberman et al., 2015). When 16-year-old Fatima left the group, Ingrid suggested that everyone write a sentence on a postcard about how Fatima had inspired them. Another child asked if a therapist could read the messages aloud. This has since become a cherished ritual, and children often smile proudly when reminded that this tradition originated from their group.

In cases where children also attend individual therapy sessions, careful coordination between group and individual contexts is essential. Discussions about what can be shared in the group are held with the child to ensure comfort and boundaries. For example, Amir has found it easier to share traumatic memories individually, but he has experienced the most significant reduction in shame and a stronger sense of belonging in the group setting. Therefore, we discuss how his memories might be shared safely within the group. Alternatively, if a sensitive topic overwhelms a child in a group session, we acknowledge that it will be addressed individually, assuring the group that their peer will receive support after the session. If, for instance, a child repeatedly expresses feeling distressed at school, this may be mentioned in network meetings with the school.

Each group session concludes with a message to the parents. One therapist writes while the group suggests content and tone. For some children, this message pre-empts further questions, while for others, it opens opportunities for discussion at home. Sometimes, it serves as a direct request. For instance, Amir once asked, "Maria, could you write that even when someone grows up and seems capable, they might still need a long hug from their mom and to hear that she's proud of them?"

Working with a co-therapist in group sessions enables therapists to mentalize each other and ensures continuity of the group process. This collaboration is essential for managing the emotional impact of trauma stories. During sessions, co-therapists model mentalizing dialogue, supporting each other through misunderstandings or uncertainties. This also provides an opportunity to demonstrate that therapists benefit from one another's perspectives and are not infallible (Karterud, 2015). Working together allows one therapist to engage with a child while the other monitors group dynamics. After each session, therapists debrief: "How did you feel during the group today? Was there something that affected you? What about now?" This reflection helps therapists mentalize themselves and each other, making implicit responses explicit. This process allows them to remain close to the trauma shared in the group while maintaining the necessary psychological distance for their own well-being.

Therapeutic interventions adapted to the children's developmental level

Our interventions are designed to align with each child's developmental stage, especially in terms of their mentalizing capacities. In our group, which spans a broad age range (8–16 years), the developmental needs vary significantly, making it crucial to use interventions adapted to different levels of mentalizing.

Attention regulation interventions

As therapists, we set up both the physical and psychological framework and boundaries for the group. When group boundaries or other insecurities come up, we are responsible for acknowledging these moments and collaboratively exploring their meaning with the group. In our group, managing attention regulation is central. When a child becomes restless or struggles to focus, it can disrupt the entire group. For instance, when Ingrid looked at her phone during a session (contrary to the group's decision to keep phones off), the therapist addressed this openly by asking if others had also broken group rules before. This brought laughter and helped lighten the atmosphere, allowing group members to share similar experiences. The other therapist then invited everyone to reflect on how Ingrid's behaviour might impact others and to consider the thoughts or feelings that might explain her actions. For children who have lived with domestic violence, this mentalizing process is crucial, helping them learn safe ways to express differing perspectives without conflict.

We also enhance group safety with predictable routines for starting and ending sessions. Predictable structures are especially important for children with developmental trauma, who may find unpredictability triggering. We begin each session by noting any absentees, followed by a check-in activity where children mark their mood on a chart. They may share anything they want the group to address, promoting self-awareness and insight into others' mental states, while also reducing misinterpretations. The therapists also participate, modelling openness by briefly sharing their own mental state, such as feeling tired after a long day, so children don't mistakenly assume it's directed at them. After reflecting on the group's progress, we end with another check-in to see how everyone is feeling, creating a chance to express how the session affected them.

Having small rituals, activities, or games that foster joint attention is crucial. The key focus areas include rhythm, structure, and the sense of being together (we-mode). In our group, we use many small games and rituals as interventions, especially when there is tension or unease among the group. For example, we might close our eyes and try to clap our hands at the same time. We stand in a circle, extend one arm straight toward the centre, and place the other arm in the opposite direction, forming a star. We then swing the outside arm toward the front hand for a joint clap. Success only happens when we synchronize our pace. This often leads to laughter when we fail, and we repeat it several times before succeeding. When the group finally succeeds, it's met with great joy. For Amir, playing in the group is something he highlights when we discuss his feelings about being part of it. Once, an older girl in the group said, "It's easier to cry in the group because we laugh so much together." Amir had been worried about his inability to cry for many years, and he often quoted her when we talked about the importance of play.

Group sessions are longer than individual ones, lasting 2½ hours. For many children, it can be difficult to sit still for that long, especially when the topics are emotionally challenging. Therefore, it's crucial to incorporate activities that activate the body. One of our favourite activities is where we all act out different emotions, and sometimes we try to guess what emotion the bodies are expressing. In another playful activity, we divide the group into two teams and the room into two halves. The teams try to throw as many softballs as possible to the other side of the room, aiming to clear their own half. The softballs have questions written on them. A timer is set for one minute, and after the play, the therapist checks in with the children to discuss what they thought and felt. Each team then picks a softball and asks the other team the question on the ball. In our group, we never count the balls because the goal is the process and the fun of the activity, not the outcome. When a child struggles with attention regulation, they can sit next to the therapist for additional support. The therapist may help regulate the child by gently placing a hand on their shoulder or co-regulating their breath.

Affect regulation interventions

Experiencing developmental trauma is often linked to difficulties with affect regulation. In a group where vulnerable topics are prioritized, it can seem inevitable that powerful emotions will rise, and without support, the children may risk becoming overwhelmed. Therefore, we aim to regulate emotions by creating awareness and engaging with all kinds of emotions through play.

Naming the level of affect and identifying the emotion can help with regulation. The therapists explicitly highlight affect regulation as it occurs during group sessions and encourage the children to talk about their experiences in the group. This includes noticing when there is a need to regulate emotions by shifting topics or introducing a new game that might trigger different feelings. For example, we often say to Ingrid, "When I look at you, Ingrid, I'm unsure if you're present or if your mind has drifted away. It's hard for me to guess what's going on inside you. Is it OK if I ask the group if they have any ideas about what might be happening inside you? Maybe they're better at guessing?" Similarly, we might ask Amir, "I notice your foot tapping; I wonder if it's telling us that this topic feels a bit overwhelming, or is the message something else? Which of your favourite games do you think would help the most right now?" These conversations give the children valuable experiences in becoming more aware of how their bodies reflect emotions and tension, and what they can do to regulate their feelings.

Focusing on affect regulation involves allowing a range of emotions in the group. When the level of safety allows it, we encourage the children to feel and express intense emotions, providing them with the opportunity to explore regulation strategies in the group. This approach is preferred over down-regulating emotions in an attempt to keep things "calm". For example, in an emotional expression game, we may support over-regulated children by "turning up the volume" of emotions, allowing them to experiment and experience that it's safe to feel these emotions and manage them with the support of the therapist and peers.

One of our regulating games involves passing a ball shaped like a human heart between group members, while expressing different emotions such as sadness, anxiety, happiness, silliness, boredom, and so on. If it's deemed relevant and safe, the emotional intensity can be increased by asking the children to throw the ball as if they felt aggression, or even violence. This may provoke laughter or discomfort, but it can also help children confront real feelings of aggression in the moment. During one game, Amir connected with his feelings of aggression; his eyes darkened, and the therapist mirrored this by saying, "It almost looks like you're not playing anymore, Amir. I get the sense that you're really feeling aggression." Amir responded, "Yes! I hate him." The therapist then asked, "OK, so you feel hate and aggression?" Amir replied, "Yes, and I hate feeling it!" The therapist responded, "Oh dear, Amir, you feel hate, but you also hate feeling it. What a powerful statement! I'm sure you have very good reasons for feeling what you feel." The therapist then turned to the group and asked, "Does anyone else recognize this feeling, or find it uncomfortable, or even hate feeling aggressive?" Almost all the children responded affirmatively. We then continued with less intense emotions, and later in the same session, we revisited the topic of aggression. We thanked Amir for feeling and showing his aggression and for sharing his thoughts with us, inviting the group to reflect on a subject that is very important for children who have experienced violence in their families.

Explicit mentalizing interventions (and recognizing non-mentalizing)

Mentalizing begets mentalizing, and within the context of a group, mentalizing is often close at hand. In the group, some children are less affected by a topic than others, which can help facilitate the mentalizing process. However, the group itself is not a safeguard against non-mentalizing – on the contrary, non-mentalizing can be contagious among group members. The group therapist must focus on engaging the children in mentalizing while also being ready to intervene when non-mentalizing occurs. When mentalizing fails, and children become overwhelmed, the need for a caring and supportive approach becomes even more important, both for the child experiencing non-mentalizing and for the rest of the group.

We introduce games and activities aimed at enhancing the mentalizing of both the group members' own life events and those of others, in the here and now. Mentalizing interventions helped Ingrid connect her inside with her outside. In one of our group activities, we explored different emotions – how they feel and how they manifest externally at varying intensities. We took pictures of the children expressing emotions at different levels of intensity, printed them out, and turned them into a guessing puzzle game. The group then had to work together to arrange the pictures in order, from the lowest to the highest emotional intensity. When it was Ingrid's turn, she quietly observed while the others struggled to guess the intensity of her expression. They found it easy to identify the most extreme expressions, but they had difficulty distinguishing the subtler ones. Ingrid tried to help, but when she looked at the pictures of her own expressions, she too had trouble sorting them in the right order. This led to a discussion about the difference between her internal experience and her external expression - being misunderstood, having teachers overlook her strong emotions, and so on. During this conversation, the therapist asked the group multiple times if they had ever experienced a disconnect between their inner feelings and their outer expressions. Many children shared similar experiences, and Ingrid seemed to pay close attention. She began to mentalize how others perceive her.

In another activity, the group discussed the typical emotions, both internal and external, of different family members during times of domestic violence. This activity activates various dimensions of mentalizing. The children might begin more cognitively, but affect can rise as the topics connect with their vulnerabilities. The activity also activates the dimensions of both internal and external mentalization, as we discuss how emotions are both felt inside and expressed outwardly, and both self- and other-mentalization, as we reflect on how different family members may feel, listen to one another, and think about their own emotions.

The next step involves selecting a number of emotions equal to the number of group members minus two. Two members (including the therapists if necessary) leave the room, and the rest of the group assigns the emotions to themselves. When the two members return, they must collaborate to guess the emotions being expressed. This approach offers several mentalizing benefits: it avoids a child being left alone if the task becomes difficult, encourages collaboration and shared thinking before making guesses, and increases thoughtfulness and mentalizing. Additionally, stepping outside the room provides an opportunity for two children to experience "we-ness" as they work together, especially if there is a new child who has been looking toward another member; sending them out together can help increase their cohesion. For Ingrid, these activities created a light, playful atmosphere that allowed her to laugh and smile during group sessions, which were otherwise focused on serious and vulnerable topics. Ingrid noticed that when she expressed sadness, her emotions were guessed correctly on the first try. She also realized that when she acted out sadness, she would quickly feel genuinely sad, something that didn't happen as easily with other emotions. "It's like my body knows this feeling too well", she said. We gently supported Ingrid in reflecting on her relationship with sadness – how it had been a significant part of her life – and acknowledged that it was difficult for everyone in the group to read the mental states behind her sad expression.

For Ingrid, it was especially helpful to recognize the difference between her internal feelings and what others could see externally. Several children in the group could relate to this experience, and one boy shared how he had learned to hide his true emotions because expressing them could lead to violence. Many children identified with the need to mask their emotions behind a facade. For Ingrid, it was valuable to hear that she wasn't alone in these experiences. She seemed to pay close attention to the older children as they shared their own struggles. At one point, she even smiled, and a younger boy remarked, "Now I can see you're happy", causing the whole group, including Ingrid, to chuckle.

These discussions became a recurring focus in subsequent group sessions. When Ingrid needed to express emotions other than sadness, the group supported her by offering suggestions for how she could express anger. They encouraged her to think about something that made her angry to help bring the feeling to the surface and suggested she "walk the anger" before showing it in her facial expression. When the group successfully guessed Ingrid's expression of anger, everyone celebrated and validated her. Through these activities, Ingrid's ability to mentalize herself deepened, and the group learned to better understand and support her emotional expressions.

A final word about Ingrid and Amir

Mentalization-based group treatment with peers provided Ingrid and Amir with profound experiences that are challenging to achieve in individual therapy. For Ingrid, the group setting allowed her to actively mentalize across the dimensions of internal–external and self–other, helping her see herself through others' eyes and fostering significant personal growth. Amir, too, found safety in sharing traumatic memories with the group and was able to explore these experiences and their effects on his life. He received affirming support from both peers and therapists, reinforcing that the violence he experienced was not his fault.

Both Ingrid and Amir felt deeply validated by their peers – an acknowledgment far more impactful than that of a therapist alone. Being part of a group, knowing they could return to share and mentalize difficult life events, created a sense of belonging and safety that was vital for both. For Ingrid, group therapy facilitated a renewed trust in herself and in others, allowing her to reconnect with her inner emotions. Amir's severe flashbacks diminished, enabling him to let go of his fear of inheriting his father's violence and instead embrace his own positive relational qualities.

Note

1 A group that takes in new members when the group is estimated to be ready. In this case, the group size has varied between 6 and 14 members during the 5 years it has lasted.

References

Asen, E. & Scholz, M. (2010). *Multi-family therapy: Concepts and techniques*. Routledge.

Graham-Bermann, S. A. & Levendosky, A. A. (2011). *How intimate partner violence affects children: Developmental research, case studies, and evidence-based intervention*. American Psychological Association.

Karterud, S. (2015). *Mentalization-based group therapy (MBT-G): A theoretical, clinical, and research manual*. Oxford University Press.

Lieberman, A., Ippen, C. G., & Van Horn, P. (2015). *Don't hit my mommy: A manual for child-parent psychotherapy with young children exposed to violence and other trauma*. Zero to Three.

Midgley, N., Ensink, K., Lindqvist, K., Malberg, N., & Muller, N. (2017). *Mentalization-based treatment for children: A time-limited approach*. American Psychological Association.

Muller, N. & Dwyer-Hall, H. (2021). MBT-A group therapy with adolescents with emerging personality disorders. In T. Rossouw, M. Wiwe, & I. Vrouva (eds), *Mentalization-based treatment for adolescents: A practical treatment guide*. Routledge.

Steinvig, R. (2022). Sammen om Børnene – én familie ad gangen. www.familieudvikling.dk/stemmer-fra-skilsmisseland/.

Vliegen, N., Tang, E., Midgley, N., Luyten, P., & Fonagy, P. (2023). *Therapeutic work for children with complex trauma: A three-track psychodynamic approach*. Routledge.

Part IV

Work with parents, carers, and the systems around traumatized children

Chapter 9

Working with traumatized children and parents together

The case of Sara

Saara Salo

Introduction: working with the whole family in the context of trauma

The decision to start working with both the parents and the child together in the context of trauma is not easy. When the child has been exposed to traumatic events such as seeing parental couple violence, it's pivotal to assess not only the child's individual needs for felt safety but also the child's needs for processing the events away from the parents. Sadly, the clinical picture is often more complex when working with these families. The question is seldom about processing only individual traumatic events but more often an accumulation of negative events in the family life, parental incapability of handling daily stress, emotional disengagement, and lack of safety which sometimes escalates into violence. From the child's perspective, the therapeutic task is then to mentalize the child's history in their family; what have the emotional conditions been like, what has the child internalized about their family relations and how has the child been able to develop emotionally.

From the parental perspective, understanding their background is equally important. Parents may bring their own (trauma) histories, psychiatric problems, and substance abuse issues to their current family. Insecure adult attachment may lead to mistrust in a couple's relationship, and adverse childhood experiences may result in the loss of affect regulation during even normal daily hassles related to parenting a young child. Thus, starting a mentalization-based intervention and deciding which family members are present in the therapeutic sessions requires doing a thorough case analysis and considering the goals of the process and individual family members' capability and feeling of safety in terms of their participation. The assessment phase can comprise different methods and approaches. It is important to consider both the child's and parents' perspectives and their needs separately, as well as considering the systemic perspective; how can we best help this family to heal when they are motivated to stay together.

In my work as a mentalization-based family psychotherapist and clinical psychologist this is a question that often comes to my therapy room, especially

DOI: 10.4324/9781032713441-14

when working with younger children. Parents and parenting quality are so important for a young child's healthy emotional development and healing from traumatic events that my goal is always to include them as much as possible. Starting from the question, "why was this child/family referred to me?", I use different kinds of approaches and methods to assess the structure and current emotional engagement between family members. In this work, I try to get a picture of the parents' level of reflectiveness about the situation, and about themselves as parents and about this child. Also, individually meeting the child and getting an understanding of their unique developmental profile, emotional coping styles and level of trust in adults are all important parts of my assessment. Hence, this phase might involve using interviews, video analyses, or just observing and listening to what the family brings to the first sessions. Through these initial meetings, I try to get a picture of the nature of the trauma as well as the most important goal of the treatment. Only after this process, will I decide whether to move into a process of family-based mentalizing work.

In the context of trauma, the decision of involving the whole family needs to be carefully considered. When the trauma is acute or family members (or some of them) show a low threshold for processing the trauma situation(s) it may be best to start with a parallel process, working with the child and parent (s) separately. It is not always easy to clinically decide the potential vulnerabilities within the child or the parents. Sometimes it becomes evident, when initially meeting and interviewing the child and the parents, that the family members may still become easily triggered, showing for example many trauma-related symptoms such as losing emotional control through getting angry or dissociating. However, many traumatized parents may have only a partial loss of their mentalizing capacity. Emotional regulation refers to all processes responsible for monitoring, evaluating, and modifying emotional reactions (Thompson & Meyer, 2007). This may include parent or child having one or two strong affect expressions or withdrawals from connection in the initial sessions. However, if the parents and/or the child are still also capable of calming down within a reasonable amount of time, with possibly some awareness of their own problems, it is possible to consider starting therapeutic work them together. Severe loses of emotional control (shouting, shutting down, acting out), denial of the family related problems, projecting and blaming the child or sometimes other people like teachers or social workers would, on the other hand, be clear contraindications for starting the process with all family members together. It is often important to be very direct in the beginning with the parents, and to ask if they are accepting and willing to work with their own emotional regulation as part of the process should such problems show up in the sessions with child. I often use therapeutic contracts in the beginning phase for this, where concrete practices such as using breathing exercises or pauses in the sessions are agreed upon.

Psychiatric illness or parental substance abuse problem are not contra-indications per se, but their effect on the parent's current functioning need to be assessed. For example, an on-going substance abuse does not usually allow for therapeutic family interventions to be effective. Parenting skills among substance abusing parents are themselves impacted by numerous chronic and inter-related problems that include medical health problems and low SES, early childhood adverse experiences in the parent's own history, and depression and other mental health problems. Together, addiction problems coupled with parental developmental trauma constitute a serious risk for a child living in these families, even without any recent traumatic events.

One area that has been shown to be particularly dysfunctional among parents with substance abuse problems is parental reflectiveness. In empirical studies, substance abusing parents typically show high levels of pre-mentalizing, i.e., having incorrect and negative beliefs about the child's intentions ("my child is teasing me deliberately") and low levels of positive mentalizing, i.e., interest and curiosity towards exploring the child's mind ("why did my child become upset?"). Instead, they often have very high (and false) certainty that their own (negatively biased) interpretation of this child's behaviour is correct (Thompson & Meyer, 2007). These reflective problems are often linked to the parents' own developmental trauma; they did not learn mentalizing skills while growing up. Even worse, when growing up with a maltreating parent, the parents' mentalizing mechanism is bound to be distorted and they are often suspicious about other's intentions as they can't trust that the even positive behaviours (such as smiling) reflect good intentions towards them Indeed, it has been suggested, that working with parental reflectiveness should therefore be the essential mechanism for change when trying to improve family connections in relation to parental substance abuse (Milligan et al., 2022). This makes MBT work also highly relevant with these families.

However, when planning MBT with parents who have substance abuse problem, taking a realistic perspective on the goals of the treatment is necessary. Sometimes the goal needs to be more in trying to help the parents to avoid negative mentalizing, such as pre-mentalizing or being too certain about what the child thinks or feels, rather than trying to directly increase their positive mentalizing, such as being interested and curious about their child's inner mental states. This realism may be especially needed when working with more complex families with both substance abuse and mental health problems. In practice, the therapist needs to be prepared to do a lot of regulative work, such as pausing and simmering down negative affect, constant efforts in building a trusting alliance and sharing their own alternative perspectives if faced with very distorted parental views on the child (pre-mentalizing).

Sometimes it may seem fruitless to work with only this side of parental reflectiveness. We therapists tend to be ambitious and strive for the more complex levels of positive mentalizing. However, as recent intervention studies highlight, it is still highly relevant from the child's perspective to lower this negative side of parental reflectiveness as it may help parents to avoid, for example, punitive child-rearing practices (Milligan et al., 2022). Taken together, when considering MBT work with parents who have substance abuse problems in their histories, doing the initial assessment of their capabilities for processing trauma, level of emotional regulation as well as their level of current parental reflectiveness is needed for setting reasonable treatment goals.

Working with Sara and her parents: how to help this family heal

In the case of 6-year-old Sara, and her mother and father, the decision to start by seeing the family together in MBT was a result of the assessment process done together with them. Sara was referred to therapy by a child psychiatric team. She was a well-developing preschooler, with no reported problems in her cognitive development. However, Sara had witnessed an incident where her parents had had a violent encounter that resulted in Sara and her mother being placed into a shelter home for a while.

Sara's parents had been together for five years before she was born. They both had substance abuse problems and together they had difficulties in managing their everyday lives, for example living with friends and not finding a stable home for themselves. When the mother became pregnant, she went into opioid replacement therapy using doctor prescribed buprenorphine, and the family ended up living all together in a mother-and-child shelter home for the first year of Sara's life. Within this program, both parents received help for their addiction problems as well as learning the new skills of being parents to a baby. The personnel in the residential setting are well-trained in enhancing early interaction as well as using various trauma approaches. Both parents described this time as a good and life-changing experience for them. Due to the previous substance use problems and related lifestyle, the father had to serve time in prison when Sara was about 2 years old, so the mother ended up taking care of Sara alone for about eight months. However, the parents were committed to staying together as a family with regular visits to prison too. When Sara's father was released, they moved to a new neighbourhood and were committed to starting a new and sober life together. Both parents recognized at the time of the first meetings with me that they still had had many unprocessed things when starting to live again as a family after the father's incarceration. They said that they did not discuss and share enough thoughts about parenting and both were also struggling to start studies or get back to work. This resulted in emotional problems within the family and escalated when Sara was about five into the violent incident that Sara had witnessed.

When considering all this information about Sara and her family, I was aware of the complexities of their situation. It was not only about one traumatic incident (violence) but also the vulnerable histories both parents would bring to the sessions. I knew that typically underneath substance use issues there are adverse early childhood experiences, difficulties in emotional regulation, and generally challenges in forming trustful relationships, including with therapists. I was thoughtful about Sara's role in all of this. It is so common that children become invisible in families with such multiple problems. On the one hand, I was wondering whether I should meet with Sara alone to give her more individual space, and on the other hand, from a systemic perspective, I was interested in seeing how her family triadic interactions were operating, and whether she was seen and heard. Hence, I decided to start with initial assessment meetings with the whole family together.

Triadic interactions in the therapy room: first meetings with the family

When first meeting the parents and Sara and hearing their history I was impressed by the level of commitment they had about making their family life work. I heard sad things, and unprocessed things too, but I also heard a genuine willingness to be together and an understanding of how things need to change from Sara's perspective. Sara was a serious girl in these first meetings, mostly sitting and drawing cats and dogs while I was discussing with her parents about why they had come to see me. Mom and Dad verbalized the reasons for coming by saying that Sara had seen a bad row between them and that this had made her scared. They said that they were sorry about it, and wanted to make things better so that everything would be safe in the family. When I was checking with Sara whether she also thought this was the reason for coming, she quietly nodded and glanced at her mom. As she didn't seem ready to do much talking, I checked with Mom whether she noticed that Sara was checking her reactions in other situations as well. Mom had noticed this, and I also noticed some sadness in the way she said this. When asking how Mom and Dad thought things could be better in their family life, each parent expressed slightly different goals. Mom was more talkative, and she sometimes seemed to express her opinion strongly while talking over Dad. Mom had many ideas about how they should divide housework more equally, start their studies, and other practical matters. I noticed that although Dad seemingly agreed, he looked a bit withdrawn. Another observation was that Sara's mom gave a lot of instructions to Sara, what to draw, where to put her pencils, where to get more paper etc. It seemed as if Mom was monitoring both Sara and Dad, as if trying to keep things under control by proactively talking and giving many instructions. It seemed a bit overcontrolling from Sara's and Dad's perspective. There was also one moment when Mom interrupted when Sara was trying to show her picture to Dad by asking to see it first.

As a mentalizing-based therapist, I was observing and noticing a triadic pattern which seemed very understandable given the parental background and the incident of violence. A genuine need to heal together, but also a lot of stress. It seemed that Mom needed to control both Dad and possibly Sara's relationship with Dad; while Sara was very cautious, holding back a lot in this session. I gently verbalized some of my observations at the end of the session, to check whether anyone else had picked up on the underlying tensions in the room. My impression was that Dad gave me the first genuine eye contact, and a little smile after this. As I didn't want to pressure them into forming any quick-fix goals for therapy, I suggested that we should just get to know each other better in the upcoming sessions through talking, and maybe playing together. I talked about good moments of being together, and how important they are to create a sense of safety and trust. I also asked both parents to focus on Sara next week and tell me a little bit about what they thought Sara especially had liked doing the next week. This focus on positive encounters seemed particularly important with this family. I had a sense of tension and even fearfulness from Sara in my therapy room, so I wanted her to know that I would not only be talking about negative things but that we also had other goals here.

Ghosts in the family living room: parents' attachment history

Before continuing with the family sessions, I wanted to meet with the parents without Sara. As a therapist, I needed to understand a bit better what safety and trust in attachment relationships meant for them, and what they had learned from their own attachment histories. In this parental meeting, we explored both parents' memories of their early childhood attachment relationships and how they currently thought these experiences affected their parenting of Sara. Both Mom and Dad told very similar stories – parental alcohol misuse and being left very much alone in their childhood. Mom linked her need for control to her past, saying that this was her way of trying to feel safe. Dad talked about difficulties in sharing his thoughts and needs and acknowledged that his way of coping was to shut down, to freeze. They told me that the one big reason for them wanting to stay together and to fall in love in the beginning was that they felt that the other one was able to understand what it means to a child to be living without safety. When talking about this, Mom was crying and she said she felt so bad that despite this very intention they had ended up creating a lack of safety for Sara. Dad agreed on this and started to talk about his guilt. I interrupted here, as I wanted to highlight at this moment that they both had such a touching and shared mentalizing of Sara's perspective. When parents themselves are developmentally traumatized, it's very hard work to keep on fighting the ghosts coming from the nursery who are haunting not only the parenting but also the couple's relationship. We talked about grief and about how hard it had been for them as an adult couple to keep on supporting each other through the battles of substance abuse and Dad being away in prison. No one had modelled to them the skills of expressing their own needs, particularly when feeling distressed. There is a place for guilt and owing responsibility for one's actions, I explained, but it is also important to recognize the vicious pattern they had been repeating in their relationship, not sharing deeper attachment needs. When I asked how they felt about this session, Mom said that for her it was very important to hear Dad talk more about his background and reasons for resorting to violence (which had only happened this one time). Dad said that for him the battle was to accept who he is, but also to try to believe that there are good things in him and that he could overcome his demons.

As a therapist, I was touched by the openness and capacity for sharing thoughts and emotions underlying their current parenting of Sara. What was also important for me, was that both parents were able to nonverbally connect with me. Even when talking about difficult past things, they had eye contact with me and I did not notice any unusual signs of bodily stress (such as heavy breathing, change in the skin colour etc). The expressed emotions (such as Mom crying) seemed appropriate and genuine even when she was not able to express with so many words about her nor Sara's feelings related to family trauma. Nevertheless, both parents showed not only cognitive insightfulness but also some genuine emotional understanding of their situations. Both parents had been working in a psychotherapeutically oriented group for substance-abusing parents for years, and I was guessing that this previous work showed here. I felt safe in continuing with family sessions.

When starting to plan MBT in the context of trauma, paying attention to nonverbal communication in the initial meetings is especially important. Implicit mentalizing, being able to attune and responds sensitively to others within a family at a nonverbal level, may provide important sources for making the decision to start to work with the whole family as well as help in formulating therapeutic goals. Thus, paying particular attention to bodily symptoms, such as the child becoming hypervigilant and/or freezing in the first family meetings, parent (or both of them) losing concentration, not monitoring how and what they speak in front of the child (such as excessive self-blame) becomes important. Other things to observe may be hostility, in the form of cold silence or becoming easily irritated by the child and/or intrusiveness, e.g., handling the child in abrupt ways. When many of these emotionally insensitive forms of interacting nonverbally with the child are present, it may be absolutely necessary to start with individual family members of help them in their emotional regulation trough trauma-related interventions before starting a MBT intervention. However, when there is a clinical sense that especially the parents have motivation and reasonable understanding of their own emotional reactions there are still clear benefits of using the whole family approach.

MBT with the family: why is Sara afraid?

In the following sessions, I often started the meeting with some attachment-based activities and games. I wanted to signal to Sara that this room was safe, there was no pressure to talk about hard things and that her parents wanted to be there with her and have a good connection. I also wanted to help the family members to connect on implicit, nonverbal level. When working in the context of trauma and fear, many reactions to other people become autonomically triggered, such as turning away, avoiding touch, etc. So my goal was to help the family members connect through this preverbal level of synchrony and reciprocity – the very underpinnings of felt safety in human connections. We played with soap bubbles, I made a handprint of all of them and we looked for similarities and differences in their physical appearances. My goal was to help the family just to pause and look at each other with openness and curiosity. During these activities Sara became much livelier, she laughed and showed a lot of initiative, especially towards her Dad. Building on this, I made a leap from this implicit mentalizing towards more explicit mentalizing: I started to notice and name these positive interactions and we had a discussion with emotion cards (little cards with different emotions drawn into them) about how they make each other feel when having a nice time together.

Also using the emotion cards, we started to explore all kinds of emotions: sad, angry, and fearful. What kinds of things make people in a family feel these feelings and how can other members then help? I asked Mom and Dad to share if they had felt these negative emotions and what had helped them to recover. I also asked Sara if she had felt any of these feelings, and she nodded and showed a fearful picture. As she didn't want to talk more about it, I went on to ask Mom and Dad if they could think about why and when Sara might have been afraid. Dad took the initiative, and he said that he thought it must have been very frightening for Sara when Mom and Dad fought. I asked Mom if she also thought this and she agreed. When I asked if had they ever talked about this with Sara, they said they had, but Mom added that she didn't think they ever talked about why that kind of situation happened. Sara looked at Mom at this point with a very serious look in her eyes. I joined in and said that that kind of a situation would be so frightening for any child and even adults, and it's good to talk about it so that everyone could be sure it wouldn't happen again. I asked Dad if he could say a little bit about what he thinks now, looking back at that moment. Dad said that he must have been very angry at that moment and what he had learned since is that adults should always be able to talk when they feel anger, and that he was very sorry he had acted out. At this point, Sara ducked down behind the sofa, but she was still listening. I asked Mom what she thought here and now hearing Dad's thoughts, and Mom said that she agreed with Sara, it was very, very frightening, and she was so happy that Mom and Dad are finally able to talk about it. She also said she wasn't afraid anymore. Sara looked at Mom, and Mom repeated this to Sara, who was hugging Mom intensely at this point.

At the end of the session, I initiated a discussion with the parents about how they could know if Sara might be experiencing fear in their everyday life, whether or not related to anything that had happened in the past. Mom was wondering aloud whether Sara could say anything and Dad said that it could also be the parents actively checking in, especially if Sara was quiet or with-drawn. At the end of this session for me as a therapist, I felt like we had opened the closed bag and that it had been ok to do so. I was also very tired myself and felt like I had to be very careful with anything that I said. I needed supervision after this session, and I had a very helpful discussion with my supervisor about my feelings and how to use them in the upcoming sessions. The main message was as I recall it: that fear is contagious. We all as human beings resonate with fear, it brings up our basic survivor instincts. To not give in to fear, and to be able to maintain a mentalizing stance is extremely hard. One would like to take a bag and shove this emotion of fear and everything related to it there. But the only way is to share and to take a perspective on it. Otherwise, the fearful state of mind will continue to colour everyday interactions.

Mother's need for control and father's helplessness

The atmosphere in the following sessions was lighter. Sara came in smiling and she was eager to start. When checking how things were at home, they talked about a nice weekend trip together. When I asked whether they had had any concerns, Dad initiated a discussion about his need to take a more active role in the home, taking care of Sara as well as participating in every-day parental decision-making. Mom interrupted and said in an irritated tone that she was the one who had to take care of everything, otherwise nothing would work. I noticed a worried look on Sara's face and paused the discus-sion, using my own need for clarification as the reason for doing so. I won-dered if we were discussing something important here and whether we should pause and explore a bit deeper? I asked if this was the pattern the parents had mentioned in previous discussions, where there is some kind of imbalance between them that caused negative feelings in the family. Since Mom was upset, I also moved closer to her, touched her gently, and asked Dad to explain what was on his mind when he made his comment. I also turned to Sara and said that sometimes it can be so worrying when parents don't agree but it's ok to discuss it here. These interventions seemed to work, and Sara's parents started to share their thoughts more calmly, Mom saying that she often tended to want to keep things "under control". This technique is called "therapist using herself" and in MBT with families it means that we can use our own emotions as examples to help parents to understand what is going on. Here I used my own uncertainty about Sara's affective expression to help parents also to pause and start processing it more deeply.

For the rest of this session, we focused on a recent situation at home, where there had been a row between the parents about who was taking Sara to bed. Starting with Sara, I asked if she remembered that evening and if she could tell or show me from the emotions cards we were using how it had been for her? She said in a quiet voice that Mom and Dad had been shouting, and she pointed to a picture of fear. I verbalized this emotion and commented how it must be frightening to hear her parents arguing. She nodded with a sad look. Turning back to her parents, who also looked sad, I highlighted how important it was for Sara or any child to tell to their parents how they feel, reminding them that this was the very reason why we were here in this therapy together. Mom – looking relieved – said that it was so sad to hear this and turned to hug Sara. Dad also moved closer to Sara and Mom. I wondered, if it would be good to know what Mom and Dad were thinking before the row, and if we could ask them to share a bit about this? Sara agreed with a nod. Mom said that she wanted to keep things under control and that she felt unsupported at that moment. I noted the times when she had had to take care of things on her own and turned to Dad to check what his thoughts were. Dad turned to Mom and said, "I'm here now". The moment was emotional and I asked Dad to repeat it to Mom and Sara. When I asked Dad how he felt in those evening situations, he said that he felt helpless, he didn't know what to do and how to help Mom. For Mom, this was a surprising feeling, and she said that for her, Dad often looked withdrawn in those situations as if uninterested. I asked if it would make sense to check with each other how they were feeling in those situations, since often the surface behaviours are not the same as internal feelings. We ended up with Sara drawing a family picture of everyone writing and drawing how they all felt inside with each other guessing what the feelings were. They all had positive feelings at the end of this session, but the interesting part was that it was still not easy to guess completely right. This reflects the fact that mentalizing does not have to be perfect, and never is. For many parents, as for Sara's parents, they have the expectation for themselves that they should understand their child perfectly. Through this exercise we got to talk about the fact that this is actually impossible, but also that it does not matter. What matters is the checking and being constantly curious: "Did I get it right?" Children and other family members will correct us if not!

In these sessions, I needed to use many interventions from the MBT model. Regarding keeping the mentalizing stance, I had to intervene to interrupt non-mentalizing, which I did by moving closer and also touching the parents. I mentioned earlier touching Mom, but I also touched Dad a couple of times. Parents, especially traumatized parents, are very different with regards how much touch and other physical closeness they need and tolerate. With some parents I have the feeling right from the start of the need to create a bit more physical space between me and them, and also avoiding using a lot of movement or sudden movements (certainly the same consideration applies to traumatized children too). With Sara's parents, however, these small moments of being there close to them and daring to share a very basic human connection was very natural and well received. Also, it seemed helpful to use my own need for clarification to help the parents to pause and reflect more. There was also room for practising the mentalizing loop, in trying to go over a typical vicious pattern and trying to explore more deeply what was going on there. When working with traumatized families, it is often about quick reactions, and over-control is a very understandable strategy for dealing with high arousal and fear. Getting some new insights and potentially a small corrective moment from the Dad, by him saying he was here now, may have helped in getting out of the negative relational patterns.

Sara starts to play

There was a change in Sara's behaviour in the following sessions. She started to take dolls and play objects from the room and initiated play. I encouraged her parents to join in and we were all playing hide and seek with the little doll figures. Sara was hiding her doll and seemed to enjoy it when her parents were seeking her doll, often looking in the wrong places in the beginning. When her parents found her doll, the doll was sometimes happy and sometimes angry, growling at the parents. I encouraged the parents to wonder with their dolls what Sara's doll might be feeling when expressing these different emotions. I was also handed a doll, and I joined in searching for Sara's doll and helping her parents' dolls find her.

This play gave me plenty to think about with the parents. We had discussions about family members sometimes wanting to hide or be invisible when there were hard times in the family, about anger in children, and how hard it was sometimes for children to show anger to their parents. Both parents shared that they had a hard time doing this when they were little. Sara was listening to our wonderings, sitting on the floor between the parents. I felt a sense of relief in these sessions. I felt that I got to know Sara a bit better and that she was starting to reveal herself more. Looking back at the therapy videos, which I often use to help me reflect on things that have happened during the session which I may not have been aware of, I also notice myself being livelier and more active, moving and approaching various family members.

Practising and breathing

Towards the end of the therapy process, we started to meet twice a month instead of weekly. In these sessions, Sara continued to express herself through a variety of play activities, such as playing with little animal characters. She enjoyed us adults joining in the play and the play themes represented normal life events, such as going on picnics as a family. I noticed that Sara's play character often did little tricks to the parent characters, and Sara seemed to enjoy it when the parent play characters were together wondering, for example where the picnic basket had disappeared. Besides these symbolic play activities, I was also able to introduce mentalizing-based activities, such as guessing the emotion game. In this game, I gave some emotions to all of them, and they had to show them to each other without words while the others were guessing which emotion it was. It seemed to be particularly exciting when I asked them to show anger; Sara was laughing out loud when her parents showed their angry faces.

When discussing daily life, and particularly the feeling of sharing things and feeling safe, the parents noticed many positive changes. They said that Sara was not as serious as she had used to be. Her parents noted that Sara was still very attentive when they had normal discussions, to check that everything was ok. But her parents seemed to be aware of this, often also turning to Sara and telling her everything was all right. Mother noticed that keeping Sara in her mind also regulated her when she started to slip into her more controlling tendencies. We also talked about self-care, taking moments just to breathe and regulate oneself when worries and insecurities started to surface in family interactions. In one of the last sessions, we practised breathing together, holding each other's shoulders standing up, and co-regulating the breathing synchronously with each other.

After we ended, about seven months from the start and 16 sessions altogether, I met Mom and Dad in a separate meeting. Their life had stabilized in many ways. Both of them still attended their own psychotherapy group meetings – Mom was thinking about her interests in university studies and Dad had found a job. They were relieved when we shared the observations about Sara in the past few months, how she seemed more lively and able to express also more negative effects to her parents. With regards to their co-parenting and feeling safe towards each other as a couple, both parents said they felt better but also that they still had to work every day to maintain their connection. We also discussed the possibility of them continuing in couples' therapy.

Ending a therapy process is never easy. I did see and feel many positive changes in this family. More positivity in their verbal and nonverbal relations towards each other, more room and focus on Sara, and also a capability of tuning in when more problematic emotions or situations occurred in family life. I was also aware that this family might encounter many more struggles and there was a continuing need for support and follow-up. However, I also felt that the parents were open to accepting help in the future. Looking now back at the whole process, I would still do many things similarly, for example, the focus on positive encounters and playing, alongside allowing more angry or scary feelings to be explored. Retrospectively, I think now that I could have been quicker in noticing Sara's withdrawal and the underlying mental states in the sessions. My sense is now that I was careful not to upset the parents, so I may have been avoiding the most important therapeutic task a little bit. For me, this retrospective understanding was important for several reasons. First, it gave me courage in thinking about future MBT work with traumatized families. By courage, I mean the trust in myself that I will not harm anyone by approaching difficult aspects in interaction more directly. This is exactly where families need help. Children's reactions are so often the ones that easier to push aside, not to really see them. My job is to catch them, look at them together with the parents – and trust that they will not be hurt or offended by me doing so. Why would they? I am really trying to help, and to blame them. This particular insight gives me strength in being active and going towards more negative mental states, especially in children, more straightforwardly. I can trust that I will be there to support the parents.

Some reflections on MBT with families who have experienced trauma

MBT with families is different from systemic family therapy, which I used with families before being trained in MBT work. As a systemic family thera- pist, the aim of the process for me was to create a new narrative with the family and to help them to start creating more constructive ways of commu- nicating with each other when faced with traumatic situations. Using a dia- logical approach, meaning helping family members to start communicating more reciprocally with each other, the therapist aims for example to help reduce the use of blaming projection (seeing one's own unprocessed emotions and thoughts only in others). By creating a new narrative, I mean a shared (re)understanding of the family history and origins, for example through using a drawing of the family tree. In drawing of family tree we studied the relations between family members often intergenerationally to start making sense of difficult past relationships, hidden family secrets and link them to the existing family relations. The content of the discussions in sessions is to deal with the current and existing problems, but also move back in time to these parental histories. The role of the therapist is to observe and interpret this narrative, with the goal of creating a new understanding, a new and hopefully more rich and coherent narrative of the current family.

With MBT, the goal for me as a therapist is more focused and happens more in the level of processing here-and-now experiences. The focus is not to explore so much the past, but in trying to help the family to get a sense of how they perceive and mentalize each other's socioemotional cues in real life episodes (sometimes being enacted right there, in the therapy room). With this focus, I pause and rewind relational situations, and help the family members to put these implicitly mentalized interactions into words, i.e. into explicitly worded understandings (or, of course, misunderstandings) of each other. By focusing on these short, enacted episodes, we try together with the family to get new perspectives (how family members perceive the same situation differ- ently), and deepen the emotional and cognitive understanding of both oneself as well that of the others. The therapist's role is very active; pausing, asking and checking the perspectives of different family members and using reflective questions, helping the family to start looking beneath behaviours, to what is actually happening in the minds of each other. With regards to moving back and forth in time in the sessions, I know about the parental history, and their level of reflectiveness in processing their past significant relationships, but in the session we stay more in the current moment, and we don't work on the interpretative (also therapist-led) level.

Taken together, the use of the MBT model brought me important things that differ somewhat from traditional systemic therapy and that I also feel are especially important with traumatized families. First, the MBT stance is hopeful as I stay in the present, visible relationships and look more towards the future rather than exploring the difficult past. Second, MBT is regulating for traumatized families who often get triggered, lose their internal affective control and, importantly, insight about others in the family. Regulation is present in the active and intervening role of the therapist. For example, my job is to interrupt non-mentalizing and simmer down difficult emotions if they should surface, or to guide the socioemotional attention to other family members when there is the risk of dropping into one's own difficult emotions, I might do this by using touch-based or emotional regulative active techniques. Third, MBT helps to create safety and alliance with traumatized families. The MBT therapist is always trying to be in the not-knowing stance, modelling interest and curiosity towards the family but not trying to take the expert position of offering the kind of interpretations which tell the family what they are "really" thinking. Alliance is difficult to achieve with parents who have learned not to trust others, including professionals who try to help them. By being open, inviting the family to share their own thoughts rather than offering yours, is one way of saying: "I am not threatening your autonomy and trying to control you". One particular way of creating this trust is to pay attention to nonverbal and embodied aspects of the session, such as where we sit, whether I move around as a therapist to make connection etc. This is also true when we have misunderstandings as a therapist. It's very much an MBT stance to notice the break-downs in communication and take responsibility for correcting these moments. Sometimes this also involves the embodied side of the session, for example noticing that I sit too close or too far away. This is a new experience for many traumatized parents who have often been blamed themselves when things go wrong.

One of the biggest clinical reasons for me to work with a whole family in the context of trauma is to be able to help in making these nonverbal interactions visible and more understandable. When working with only the child or with only the parents we are working on a representational or episodic memory level of family interactions. We don't really see what is happening, especially at the nonverbal, implicit level. In *in vivo* situations, being able to be there with the family, holding and pausing the situation, may give the family a real emotionally corrective experience. I believe that its through these shared moments of being able to repair, to be able to help the parents gain more emotional regulation and to help the child to re-orient towards the parents we are really giving them hope and tools in their real-life situations. They are living together and these kinds of negative, non-mentalizing cycles are inevitably present in their everyday lives. If we, as therapists, are not experiencing them together with them, then who is?

The last time I met Sara's family was at a Christmas party last year. It was a gathering for all clients at the outpatient unit of the mother-and-child shelter who had participated in treatment programs there. Sara was now an 8-year-old, shy, sweet girl who loved horses. She remembered me and came to greet me at the party. Mom was studying developmental sciences at the university and Dad was working. The reunion was touching, as Sara made immediate warm contact with me and suggested that we play with bubbles. This made Mom and Dad laugh, and they said they still did this sometimes as a family.

You don't always hear from your therapy patients after the work ends. I was grateful for this encounter. It was also hopeful. When working in the context of trauma and complex life histories, it's good to be reminded about the possibilities for change. All families deserve help – maybe in different ways and focusing sometimes on different family members, but 'whole family' really is our secure base. Nurturing that place through MBT work with families, using both explicit mentalizing strategies and also creating a safe place to practise new and more positive nonverbal relatedness, seemed particularly helpful with Sara's family. I wish to sincerely thank them for everything that I learned as a therapist from them.

References

Milligan, K., Rodrigues, E. R., Daari-Herman, L., & Urbanoski, K. A. (2022). Parental reflective function in substance use disorder: individual differences and intervention potential. *Current Addiction Reports*, 9 (1), 59–66.

Thompson, R. A., & Meyer, S. (2007). Socialization of emotion regulation in the family. In J. Gross (ed.), *Handbook of emotion regulation* (pp. 249–268). Guilford Press.

Chapter 10

Working with parents who have experienced adverse childhood experiences

The challenge of blocked care

Masja Juffermans and Hanneke van Aalst

Every parent has to deal with the imprint of their own history in how they care for their own children. Parents who have experienced adverse childhood experiences (ACEs), such as child abuse or abandonment, can struggle with unresolved trauma. They may have difficulty providing the best care for their child despite their desire to do so (Alink et al., 2019; Borelli et al., 2019; Weistra et al., 2025). When these parents have to cope with their child's mental health problems, they may have to deal with a double dose of parental stress, related to their traumatic history and their child's emotional difficulties (Dollberg & Hanetz-Gamliel, 2023). Sometimes these parents are inundated with trauma triggers, which blur their view of their child. This can get in the way of connecting with the child sensitively and responsively and impacts on the attachment relationship and the development of mentalizing skills and epistemic trust in the child. This heightened parental stress may further shake the parents' mentalizing skills (Dollberg & Hanetz-Gamliel, 2023). We refer to this process as "blocked care", which can lead to blocked mentalizing (Ensink et al., 2015; Ensink et al., 2016; Hughes, 2016).

In this chapter, we describe the challenges that clinicians may encounter when working with traumatized parents: through the account of work with one particular family, who agreed to us writing about them, whose names and some details have been changed for confidentiality. In describing the case, we explore four key pillars:

1 building epistemic trust;
2 how to work with parents who have suppressed their own feelings and are afraid of overwhelming feelings related to traumatic experiences;
3 blocked care; and
4 working towards sustainable change.

Case introduction

Mr Brown and Mrs Rose, a separated couple, came into our Child and Adolescent Mental Health Service (CAHMS). They both had several Adverse

DOI: 10.4324/9781032713441-15

Childhood Experiences (ACEs) in their early lives and there had been a violent relationship when they were together. Their daughter Sharon (10 years old) was referred by social services because there was much concern about her behaviour. She was rebellious, lied, had few friends, and had low self-esteem. Sharon frequently had angry moods where she showed destructive behaviour. She either destroyed valuable items or physically harmed herself. Most of the time Sharon lived with her mother, stepfather and her older and younger brothers (13 and 2 years old). Sharon and her older brother Dylan fought a lot. She visited her father and his new partner twice a month.

Mr Brown appeared to have less concerns about Sharon's behaviour. It took several conversations with social services before he gave permission to seek help for his daughter. Sharon had previous treatment at the Medical Day-care, with a focus on behaviour change. Her parents received tips which they told the worker from social services were not very effective. Sharon also had play therapy for one and a half years, but with insufficient results, leaving the parents and Sharon with feelings of helplessness and little confidence that further therapy would work.

Our team decided to offer Sharon time-limited mentalization-based treatment (MBT), involving work with the parents alongside individual therapy for the child (Midgley et al., 2017). Two therapists were assigned to the case – one to work with Sharon, and the other to work with the parents and their new partners. After the assessment phase Sharon and her mother were seen in time-limited MBT for three "blocks" of 12 sessions – a total of thirty-six weekly sessions. They had individual sessions (45 minutes) at the same time, followed by a joint part (fifteen minutes) to talk about what they had worked on in the session. In addition to the live conversations with mother, the therapist had several online meetings with father and his partner. As part of the MBT time-limited model, we also aimed to have a joint parent–child session with mother and Sharon in session eight of each calendar, to review progress and plan the next steps. Father attended these sessions online.

Sharon and her parents needed the first twelve sessions to decrease their epistemic mistrust of us as professionals and build a relationship with the therapists. An essential aim of the second block of twelve sessions was to enhance Sharon's and the parents' attention and emotion regulation so they could respond to each other in a more flexible and attuned way. During the review meeting of the second block of 12 sessions, the therapist and the parents decided to start a third block to consolidate and generalize what had been achieved in the context of treatment. In the third block a significant amount of time was spent giving Sharon and her parents the opportunity to experience a meaningful goodbye.

Building epistemic trust and engagement with traumatized parents

Be brave, you never know what a first meeting might lead to.

(James Norbury, 2021, p. 22)

Besides making a mentalizing profile of the child and parents, another aim of the assessment phase in MBT is to get the parents engaged in the therapy process. Traumatized parents often experience epistemic mistrust or hypervigilance towards others. They do not have enough good, trustworthy experiences that allow them to open up to therapists and see them as potentially helpful. Therapies are often stopped prematurely because parents feel misunderstood and judged (Fonagy et al., 2019). It is a challenge to think about ways to help these parents connect and trust the therapist and accept help, in order to get their mentalizing and parenting back on track. Before the initial meeting with parents, a team might want to think together about what these parents might need to feel at ease and supported so they can become engaged and develop epistemic trust.

During the telephone conversation prior to the first session of Mr Brown and Ms Rose, both parents explicitly stated that a joint starting session would create too much tension, not trusting each other and not yet trusting the clinicians. Being "reasoned flexible" (Slade, 2008), the team started with individual parallel sessions and work towards joined sessions at a later stage, when epistemic trust had (hopefully) increased.

Another regulating intervention can be to ask parents whether they want to bring someone to the initial meeting to give them the emotional support they need. We asked both parents if they would like to bring their current partners, which we thought might have a positive effect on lowering their epistemic mistrust. However Mr Brown didn't come to his first appointment, explaining he couldn't make it "because he had no car". The therapist wondered if he was also avoiding this first contact. Traumatized parents have often developed a pattern of avoiding situations that might give them tension. It is a highly effective defence mechanism that is difficult to change. Father had not been involved in the previous therapies and the therapist didn't want this pattern to be repeated. He was important for the MBT therapy, knowing that Sharon visited him twice a month on weekends and he was an important person to her.

The therapist discussed the situation in her team and they decided to meet with father online.

In the first appointment, he was very clear: he would be cooperative because he wanted the best for his daughter, but he didn't require any help himself. His previous experiences were that therapists only portrayed him as the father who caused his daughter's problems. He believed he had been mistreated. Mr Brown spoke loudly and firmly, often using harsh statements. He appeared to be in a "psychic equivalence" mode, convinced of his perspective on everything. The therapist felt a bit overwhelmed and anxious in the conversation, which made it challenging for her to establish a genuine connection.

Parents in treatment are not only learners; they are also communicators. They come into therapy wanting the therapist to trust them in their view of themselves and their child (Malberg et al., 2023). Keeping this need of Mr Brown in mind, the therapist tried to slow down the process by asking him about the words he used, or to be curious about the meaning of his expressions. She explained to him she wanted to understand the situation and his perspective by saying, "I think you are expressing something important here, and I want to make sure I understand what you say". But her questions didn't seem to have the effect she intended, and words didn't seem enough to build trust. She tried to validate father's feelings by saying she could imagine he may have felt tense to have his first meeting because of his former experiences. He became agitated and denied feeling tense, saying, "You don't know me".

It can be challenging to offer empathetic validation when you don't have a full understanding of the interactions and emotions. If you behave in a way that is incongruent with what you say, it can increase mistrust and decrease credibility. Mr Brown's hostile and dismissive attitude and the online contact were a real challenge for the therapist and her mentalizing capacity. Her first inclination was to not involve father in therapy. She discussed the strain on her mentalizing and her feelings towards the father with her team. Working in a team is very helpful in dealing with all these challenging processes, and not becoming powerless, mistrusting and non-mentalizing ourselves. Feeling safe and supported in a team, where reflective questions about the therapist's own assumptions and beliefs can be explored, is helpful in unravelling the implicit aspects of the relationship between the therapist and the parent and helps the therapist to stay on track (Midgley et al., 2017).

The therapist told her team about her effortless attempts to show empathy and taking Mr Brown's concerns seriously. The team thought father was frequently in a teleological mode and could be a man who might prefer action over words. The team decided to offer a home visit to Mr Brown to meet him and his family in person. He agreed to this. Knowing a home visit can result in difficult situations, the therapist asked the child therapist to come with her to ensure her own safety. The therapists drove for two hours, with the effort involved a clear sign of her genuine wish to see and understand him. Both therapists received a warm welcome from Mr Brown, who appeared to be much more relaxed when he was in the safety of his family environment, which helped him to maintain his mentalizing stance. The therapists saw a nice and warm contact between father and daughter. The therapist was now able to think about the father as someone who could communicate in a hostile way, but on the inside, he seemed to have good intentions and warm feelings towards his daughter. This appeared helpful in future interactions, as it allowed the therapists to stay curious as they tried to see the different sides of this father.

In the online conversations with Mr Brown, the therapist explicitly invited his partner each time, knowing that her presence positively affected Mr Brown's epistemic trust. During and after the sessions, the therapist was aware that epistemic trust was emerging but was still fragile. After each online session, she took a moment to reflect on the meeting and wondered what mental states she thought father was in and how these mental states affected his epistemic trust. In the appointments, she explicitly invited him to express his thoughts and feelings and talk about the interaction between him and the therapist so they could keep up the work together for the best for Sharon. With the support of his partner and the mentalizing stance of the therapist, Mr Brown was able to regulate his feelings better and talk about his history and traumas. He shared that he was a victim of domestic violence and abuse by his father. As Mr Brown became more open about his problems with his daughter and his concerns, the therapist could also support and validate him, enhancing the trust between them.

At this point the therapist wrote a letter to Mr Brown expressing her candid thoughts and emotions, which she read out loud to him and his partner. Writing and reading the letter aloud to the parents is a key moment in therapy where the therapist conveys the message: "I have seen you, what you tell me is important." It is a teleological action where the therapist shows that she and the team take time to write down their thoughts, feelings and emotions about the parents and the relationship with their child. Reading the letter out loud creates an opportunity to use ostensive cues, like using a warm tone of voice and, when culturally appropriate looking people in the eye, marking the importance of the message and making a heart-to-heart connection. Many traumatized parents are not used to people thinking about them in a caring way. It is crucial to be sincere and open about the parents' positive parenting skills and dare to discuss the problematic interactions and feelings. By relating the mentalizing profile of the parent to the present interaction with their child, the focus for therapy can be established.

In our case, both parents received a letter. Our letter to Mr Brown was as follows:

> Mr Brown, Sharon has a special place in your heart, but lately, you feel less able to understand your daughter. Mr Brown, I sense and experience that you are distrustful of counselling services. I want to express my appreciation for sharing your concerns, commitment to your daughter's therapy, and wanting to be part of the treatment process. You express your distrust clearly and intensely to the outside world, which can scare the other person off. As you have told me more about your past, I have understood that you had to learn to trust your opinion and that you needed your firm stance as a protective shield to keep you from getting hurt again. Looking beyond your behaviour, I have come to know you as a father who loves his daughter and has her best interests at heart.
>
> You told me you are a man of clear rules and agreements. This can be a strength at times of calmness and gives Sharon a lot of clarity and predictability. When tension gets high, you sometimes can become too firm, and to this firmness, Sharon responds with anger and resistance, resulting in a situation in which you are shouting at each other. This is upsetting and unsafe for both of you, and you told me you don't want

this anymore. I would like to invite you to join me in looking beyond Sharon's (challenging) behaviour, reflecting a bit more on Sharon's intentions and feelings, the same way as I did in our conversations about you. Together, we can think about why she behaves in a certain way, what Sharon needs at these moments and what you need as a father to respond to Sharon's needs. I sincerely hope I can support you in this.

In our clinical experience, many parents are touched when the letter is read out loud. This "moment of meeting" can positively impact the parent's relationship with the therapist. The mistrust was strong in Mr Brown's case, and the therapist noticed an ambivalent reaction. He recognized himself in the letter, which made him feel seen and more relaxed, but he had difficulty showing his emotions, and some distance remained palpable between them. It was, however, the start of a shared vision of the interaction between a father and his daughter.

In working with traumatized parents, epistemic trust is not built in a few sessions and will remain fragile during the therapy. For some parents it might be the first time they meet a therapist who regards them as having a mind with agency and intentionality that is worth understanding (Malberg et al., 2023).

The courage to feel again: giving parents the experience of being kept in mind

No one can see their reflection in running water.
It is only in still water that we can see.

(Taoist proverb)

After experiencing chronic trauma, the body can become a place where powerful tension is felt where symptoms related to emotion dysregulation may overwhelm parents and interfere with their ability to respond sensitively and consistently to their child (Meijer et al., 2023). Traumatized parents may have developed multiple defence mechanisms and interactional patterns in an attempt not to get overwhelmed or hurt again. Avoiding or blocking feelings is one of the defence mechanisms that are almost immediately visible in the therapy room, especially with MBT where the affect focus is one of the core elements. As MBT therapists, we can help traumatized parents connect with their (partly dissociated) inner world or become less afraid of these big tsunami-like feelings. Instead of avoiding feelings, we must help parents slow down and feel again by creating a space where parents feel seen, safe and become curious about what's underneath their water surface and what the behaviour of their children is trying to show about what is inside their child.

But how can you help to still the waters inside? A mentalizing approach, where the parents are kept in mind and heart when they feel their pain, can help parents explore how their relational past influences the way they deal with their own emotions and the relationships with their children (Malberg et al., 2023). Many parents have little experiences where they felt seen and understood, being held in mind and heart, making it very hard to pass this on to their child. We need to give the parents what the child needs and shine a light on their inner world so they can experience how it feels when you are kept in mind and how this helps regulate emotions. When the parents feel mentalized, this will open their capacity to mentalize about their child and the relationship between the parent and child.

In the assessment phase, when the therapist was working hard to engage Mr Brown, she also continued to meet separately with Mrs Rose to build epistemic trust and develop a mentalizing profile of her and Sharon. In the family session, Mrs Rose, her partner, her sons, and Sharon were all present. The family session turned out to be chaotic. Mrs Rose and her partner provided few boundaries and structure for their children, resulting in a situation in which the youngest boy threw toys across the room. At that moment, Mrs Rose seemed to be in a state of freeze. After a while, she regrouped herself and took physical action when she pulled the youngest onto her lap. She did so without verbalizing her actions or making eye contact with her son.

Mrs Rose attended the following session alone, as her partner was unable to come. She barely looked at the therapist and sat stiffly in her chair. She spoke in a soft voice with very little vitality and a tight facial expression. Mrs Rose answered the questions but showed no initiative in the conversation. The therapist noticed the distance in Mrs Rose's body language and saw she was avoiding eye contact. The therapist was curious if this was related to her actions in the previous session. She wondered if the specific way Mrs Rose's body was reacting (making herself small, avoiding meeting the eyes of the other) might be telling a story of how she has adapted her moves, posture, and tone of voice to survive earlier in her life (Odgen et al., 2020). In this beginning phase of their work together the therapist started by focusing on the here and now and on giving Mrs Rose an experience of being kept in mind while she felt tense. She worked on the boundaries of the "window of tolerance", so Mrs Rose could see that feelings can come and go. The therapist slowed down the pace of the conversation and became aware of her own body and the tension she felt. After observing her own bodily state, the therapist sat back so she felt the support of her chair which helped her focus on what she experienced in the relationship with this mum. She felt tension in her muscles and noticed she had become a bit cautious. In working with traumatized parents, it is helpful to remain aware of our own bodily sensations and recognize somatic transference. The therapist tried to lower the tension in the room and tried to capture Mrs Rose's attention by maintaining an open body position. She was aware that she used ostensive cues, for example by actively addressing Mrs Rose by her first name. She spoke with a warm, soothing tone to try and regulate Mrs Rose's emotions and communicate implicitly that she was safe.

The therapist tried to help Mrs Rose to become aware of her non-verbal communication by noticing and naming what was happening in the here and now and showing a general interest in her subjective experience by saying: "When I look at you, I see much tension in your face and body and I am aware I also start to feel tension inside myself". She checked her observation by asking: "Does this resonate with you? Do you feel tense?". Mother nodded. Checking facial expressions, tone of voice, body gestures and using marked mirroring with Mrs Rose by repeating her words with a slightly different emotion had the aim of showing her that the therapist was paying attention. Implicitly this gave Mrs Rose the message that the therapist took her seriously as a communicator and that she was someone worth listening to, which helped enhance her self-agency. The attention of the therapist also helped Mrs Rose to shift her attention inward asking: "Where do you feel this tension in your body, can you show it to me?". Mrs Rose moved her hand towards her chest. The therapist mirrored her movement by placing her hand on her chest to say: "OK, so you notice tension in your chest". After the therapist helped Mrs Rose connect with her emotions, she tried to clarify what range of emotions mother felt and what experiences had led to all these emotions.

Many parents who have experienced their own trauma ignore their bodies and miss the affective cues or, worse, suppress them (Malberg et al., 2023). By shifting the attention from external to internal cues, the therapist starts connecting between external bodily gestures and inner sensations. For Mrs Rose this was a new experience in which the therapist helped her approach her sensations and feelings instead of moving away from them in a dysregulated state. This experience is one from which she could draw on when the attention was shifted to her daughter and what she needed when she had (intense) emotions. Mother appeared to need many of these experiences in multiple sessions before she could pass this experience on to Sharon. This is one of the reasons that it took 36 sessions to complete the therapy.

Blocked care: how to identify patterns and break repeating cycles

We repeat what we don't repair.

(Christine Langley-Obaugh, 2023)

In working with traumatized parents, it is important to be mindful of how repeating patterns and/or traumatic events from the past impact the present, especially in the parent–child interaction. With these parents, it is sometimes about balancing to what extent you can dwell with parents on the effect of their own childhood on their parenting with their child now and providing therapy for the parents themselves (Whitefield & Midgley, 2015). Parents seem often unaware of the connections between past traumatic experiences and present feelings. Triggered emotions can surprise and overwhelm them, resulting in a breakdown in mentalization. As a therapist, it is important to be alert to these triggers and breakdowns and slow down the process when it happens. When we find ways of remaining with the parents in these emotional states, these moments are possibilities to enhance their attention and affect regulation and create a narrative from which parents can understand their feelings and behaviour. The therapist seeks to create a supportive environment that can serve as a secure base for parents, from which they can develop their capacity to provide a safe haven for their children (Malberg et al., 2023, p. 124).

An example of Mrs Rose being triggered by past traumatic experiences happened in the joint part of session 6. Sharon talked spontaneously about how things were like at home. According to Sharon, mother was often very angry and abusive. She called mother a devil who yelled at her and sometimes pushed her when she was sent to her room for punishment. Mrs Rose was overtaken by her daughter's openness, resulting in a state of freeze in which she hardly said anything. The therapists were caught off guard by Sharon's statements and the tension that was suddenly building in the room. They tried to support Sharon and mother simultaneously by saying it was brave that Sharon talked openly about her experiences, and they also acknowledged it caused a lot of tension for both. They tried to be transparent, telling mother and Sharon they wanted to take the time to explore everyone's thoughts and feelings to get an understanding of their experiences. The therapists decided to get back to this in the next session with mum.

In the days between sessions the therapists felt insecure about how they had dealt with the situation and doubted their decision to come back to the situation in the following session. They were worried about how mother would react to Sharon's words at home. They started to feel the need to call mother and check how she and Sharon were doing. But they decided to reflect on these needs and feelings with their team before rushing into action. The team helped restore their faith in the intervention and in mother's capacity for emotion regulation, helping them to trust that she could endure the "not knowing" until the next sessions.

In the upcoming parent session with Mrs Rose, the therapist was aware of the possibility of high emotions in the room. She had to start working on the attention regulation in the here and now before she could go back to the situation from the previous meeting. After the therapist paid attention to the present feelings, the tension in the room decreased, and mother appeared to be more relaxed and engaged. The therapist summarized what they had just discussed, conveying to Mrs Rose she had listened carefully. The therapist created a safe base for mother to work on a second level where they could explore and mentalize together about what happened in the previous session and at home afterwards.

Mrs Rose said that the sudden openness of Sharon in the previous session had triggered a painful memory of her youth when she trusted a school counsellor and told her about the sexual abuse of her brother. This resulted in an intervention where mother was taken to a crisis centre without any expla-nation. As a result, her brother was placed out of home and never returned. This had a great impact on her family for a long time, and she felt very guilty about this. She was afraid that history would repeat itself and that she would lose her daughter: "In my mind, I have always known that my past experiences would one day deceive me."

The therapist supported mother in acknowledging that this must have been a very upsetting experience, and she could imagine that it had a lot of impact on her. To understand the situation fully, she wanted to make an affective narra-tive with mother asking: "Can you tell me a bit more about what happened at the moment this memory came up?"

For Mrs Rose it wasn't easy to explain. "I experienced a range of emotions, and my mind was racing". The therapist replied: "Mm, so a range of emotions. What signals was your body giving you?" Mother said her heart started beating faster, and her face felt warm. "What were you feeling?". She felt tremendously anxious. "What were you thinking when your mind started racing?"

"They will think I am a bad mother and probably place Sharon out of the house too."

"What happened when you started thinking that?"

"I panicked, and my mind went blank. I heard Sharon making statements that were not true. I wanted to flee from the situation and never come back."

The therapist noticed that, as they were speaking, the temperature in the room started rising again. She offered empathic validation to help mother regulate her emotions saying: "It must have been awful for you to have all these feelings and think that we would judge you and see you as a bad mother. Thank you for sharing this because it helps me understand why you didn't want to come back to therapy."

After exploring the internal world of Mrs Rose, the therapist felt there was room for mother to shift her attention to her daughter and the impact this situation would have had on their relation, asking: "What happened when you went home? How did you feel about your daughter?" Mrs Rose told she was mad at Sharon on the inside but did not put her feelings into words. She became quiet and was so absorbed in her feelings of panic and her traumatic memories that she couldn't respond sensitively to Sharon (blocked care). Mrs Rose reflected on this interaction, telling the therapist this was a familiar pattern between the two of them: when Sharon falsely accused mother, she got overwhelmed and stopped being mindful of Sharon.

The therapist asked Mrs Rose what Sharon saw on the outside when she was mad. Mother started mentalizing about her daughter: "I think she can feel that I am mad, but my face looks tense?" Together, they mentalized about how confusing and unsafe this might have felt for Sharon and what she needed at these moments. Mrs Rose wanted to give more guidance to Sharon and tell her what she could and could not say. This would make it safer for mother and her daughter. She became more curious about why Sharon was making these statements. Could she be looking for guidance and boundaries, or was she seeking attention? The therapist ended the meeting by asking Mrs Rose how she had experienced this session, and if she felt judged (as she feared), or if she was leaving the room with another feeling. Mrs Rose explained that she was surprised and relieved to see and hear that the therapist didn't judge her. The therapist responded that we can all fall into certainties when experiencing painful emotions and added that she admired mother's bravery and willingness to look at her own feelings and explore other possible reactions to the therapist.

During the following session, Mrs Rose mentioned that she had been thinking a lot. She never realized that her emotions are important signals worth acknowledging and acting on. Instead of dismissing them, she wanted to take them seriously and take her daughter's feelings seriously as well. She wanted to connect more with Sharon, so she bought a book with all kinds of questions about feelings and started to read it with her. The curiosity of the therapist and the experiences of being held in times of overwhelming feelings awoke a curiosity in Mrs Rose about her and her daughter's internal world.

Working towards sustainable and meaningful change

From the beginning of therapy, therapists work with the understanding that we are only involved in the lives of our clients for a short while. So we do not just pay attention to the actual goodbye in the final sessions but also keep endings in mind from the start and adjust our attitude from the beginning. Having knowledge of attachment patterns can help us as therapists to understand how we must act and communicate and set the ground for sustained and meaningful change (Malberg et al., 2023). We have to involve the parents' network in the work as well because re-opening epistemic trust in the therapeutic context is merely one part of a process of social learning. This process needs to be supported in the parents' wider social environment for there to be any chance of a sustained, meaningful change (Fonagy & Allison, 2012).

In working with parents with an avoidant attachment style like Mr Brown, an important aim of the therapy is to re-open epistemic trust in the therapeutic context. This isn't easy because these parents are not used to learn from others and often only trusted their own opinions. In contact with these parents, it is necessary to "squeeze into the contact" to trigger their interest (Hutsebaut et al., 2023, p. 71). By enhancing joint attention, for example by inviting parents to stop and pay attention to something that has happened, parents who may usually be quite avoidant can start to register the ostensive cues which the therapist is providing and experience being taken seriously and trusted by the therapist. Then it may be possible for parents with an avoidant attachment style to gradually become more open to what we are communicating to them, which can lead to more reciprocity in the relationship. This paves a way to the "we-mode" (Fonagy et al., 2022), where through co-mentalizing, different perspectives can co-exist and mutually influence each other. From this point, parents can gain a new experience in how relationships can enrich their own perspective.

Mr Brown and the therapist had moments when they came to a shared place of thinking and feeling together and he experienced that sharing could be enriching. During the middle and final phase of therapy, the therapist and Mr Brown discussed the importance of sharing and identified which friends and family members could support him after therapy ended. Father reached out to his partner and a friend who could both provide support in times of stress and help him regain a broader perspective on his interactions with his former partner, when his mentalizing was breaking down.

When parents have a preoccupied attachment style and little self-agency, such as Mrs Rose, they can become clinging and dependent on counselling and the therapist, which can eventually lead to great uncertainty at the end of the therapy. Previously developed trauma reactions can reinforce these relational patterns. When fight-and-flight mode does not help, people may be tempted to cling to the one person who might be able to help them, in a cry for help (Fisher, 2020). Parents can repeat this trauma response in the therapeutic relationship (re-enactment). A parent's feelings of despair, powerlessness, insecurity, and dependency may tempt the therapist to take care of the parent by giving them advice or solving problems for them. However, this can lead to even more dependency and reinforce the feeling that parents cannot do it themselves. We therefore try to find a balance in providing support, but not allowing parents to lean on us too much, so we can strengthen their self-agency.

A possibility to enhance Mrs Rose's self-agency appeared in a session in the middle phase of the therapy. Mrs Rose came to therapy in a panic state. She immediately started speaking when she entered the room. Mr Brown had sent her an email saying that he wanted Sharon to move in with him. Mrs Rose was very upset and afraid she would lose her daughter. She talked quickly and chaotically, which made it difficult to understand her story. Mrs Rose asked if the therapist could call Mr Brown to tell him this would be a wrong decision that couldn't be made. The sooner, the better. The therapist noticed and named how stressed and anxious mother was. The therapist was confused by the sudden turn of events because she didn't recognize anything about it from the last conversation with Mr Brown. The therapist supported and validated mother by saying she can imagine that this is a complicated and very upsetting situation, but she didn't immediately respond to the request to call Mr Brown. She suggested they sit down on the chairs and take some time to explore together what Mrs Rose was feeling and thinking before they rushed into solutions.

The therapist noticed she was feeling a bit of mother's panic as well. Her heart was racing, and she felt tempted to speak to father about this. She decided to slow down, explore, and clarify what had touched mother so much that her mentalizing broke down, leading her to go into a teleological mode, asking her for all kinds of actions. It struck her that mother seemed to believe that the content of the email equalled reality. She seemed to have lost the belief that she had a voice in this. The therapist explored Mrs Rose's thoughts and feelings when she read the email. Mrs Rose said she immediately felt panic because of her ex-partner's firm tone in the email. She froze, felt powerless and once again at the mercy of what he wanted. It made her anxious, sad and convinced she couldn't solve it herself. The therapist supported her in how hard it must have been for Mrs Rose when she was overwhelmed by all these feelings. She explicitly shared what was on her mind:

> I can see you are upset. If I were in your shoes, I would have been startled by the firm tone of the email. I felt the need to protect you, and my first thought was to call Mr Brown as you asked me. This might have made you feel less anxious in the short run, but I don't think this will help you in the long run. If I called Mr Brown, I would have undermined your parenting skills because I have come to know you as a mother who can think about what is best for her daughter and act on it.

Instead of directly responding to Mrs Rose's request to call her ex-partner, the therapist focused on her inner strength. As a result, mother realized that she could play an important role in the process and didn't need to depend on the therapist to solve her problems. The therapist chose to share her thoughts and feelings so she and mother could come to a mutual understanding of the process between them. In this "we-mode" (Fonagy et al., 2022) the therapist and Mrs Rose engaged in joint attention, maintaining their distinct minds while acknowledging their commonalities.

Saying goodbye

A meaningful farewell creates a memory that endures.

The end of therapy should be an opportunity for the parents to revisit, re-experience and learn new ways of dealing with the emotions that arise when saying goodbye is approaching. Traumatized parents often have a lot of painful, broken relationships, fights and losses. For them, it can be challenging to end therapy in a nice way, knowing that saying goodbye activates the attachment system of the parent (Malberg et al., 2023). It is therefore helpful to think together with the team about the attachment style of the parents and the therapist and how they will influence the process of saying goodbye when therapy comes to an end.

In the work with Mr Brown it meant that the therapist kept in mind that saying goodbye during a session was new for him. He was used to ending relations abruptly and through conflict, so this could be the first time for father to say goodbye with attention. This made them think about an appropriate farewell, not too grand nor too emotional, but connected. This allowed the therapist and father to reflect on how they had experienced the therapy process and how he could use relationships, including with his current partner, in his daily life to support him.

In the process with Mrs Rose there was a bit of a surprise in the ending phase when Mrs Rose emailed the therapist to let her know that she couldn't come to the therapy anymore. She needed to work more hours because of her financial situation. The therapist was confused. She felt a bit side-lined, as if she was not important. Again, she shared the situation with her team to help her think about what might be going on here. The team explored and validated her feelings, and brought in another perspective by noticing that it might be a very positive development that Mrs Rose took the initiative to end the therapy instead of holding on to the therapist out of fear of letting go. The team also assisted her in reflecting on mother's narrative and the challenges she had faced in the sudden and disruptive endings of previous relationships. Could it be that like father, also this mother did not yet have a script for saying goodbye? Possibly, no one had ever paid attention to her in these moments. The therapist felt it was important to her and for the therapeutic process to express her need for a good ending since the therapy had been important to her. The therapist wanted to give Mrs Rose a new experience of separation with attention, with the message that she was a person worthy of saying goodbye to. She decided to call Mrs Rose and discuss her thoughts and feelings and mark their goodbye as an essential moment. The therapist's words seemed to resonate with Mrs Rose, made her feel important and helped her to realize that she wanted to say goodbye too. Together, she and the therapist managed to have several sessions where they could reflect on the treatment process, with a particular focus on the development of mother, to see herself as an agent of change.

Some reflections on working with traumatized parents

No matter how hard traumatized parents try to give their child everything they need, unintentional trauma often impacts their parenting and the parent–child interaction (Meijer et al., 2023). Promoting and restoring mentalizing skills of parents who have endured ACEs and whose children have mental health issues can serve as a protective factor for the parent, the child and the parent–child relationship (Dollberg & Hanetz-Gamliel, 2023).

In this chapter, we have tried to outline four key pillars in working with parents who have endured ACEs. Amidst all the emotions and tensions in the room, it can be quite difficult to maintain our focus during therapy. Working with traumatized parents can be an unpredictable and challenging process for the therapist. Engaging these parents in therapy takes time and involves creativity. In the case of Mrs Rose and Mr Brown reopening the epistemic trust and enhancing their attention and emotion regulation demanded a lot from the therapists and put a strain on their own mentalizing capacity. Working in a team created a nonjudgmental space where they could constantly pause and reflect on their thoughts, feelings, mentalizing collapses and recovery, and that of the parents as well. Just as the parent needs to be sufficiently regulated in order to regulate the child, the therapist has to be sufficiently aware and regulated in order to regulate and help the parent become aware of his or her past trauma and how it is linked with parenting and the child's current difficulties (Dollberg & Hanetz-Gamliel, 2023). This can sometimes motivate parents for further therapy to process these trauma's in their own trauma-therapy. When the therapist is able to do this, there is a real possibility that parents with a history of trauma themselves can be given an experience of being cared for, which in turn supports them to become the parent they truly want to be for their child.

Acknowledgements

A special thanks to the parents who worked very hard to help their daughter. Also, a very special thanks to Wendy Backx and colleagues who worked in this case.

References

Alink, L. R. A., Cyr, C., & Madigan, S. (2019). The effect of maltreatment experiences on maltreating and dysfunctional parenting: A search for mechanisms. *Development and Psychopathology*, 31 (1), 1–7. doi:10.1017/s0954579418001517.

Borelli, J. L., Cohen, C., Pettit, C., Normandin, L., Target, M., Fonagy, P., & Ensink, K. (2019). Maternal and child sexual abuse history: An intergenerational exploration of children's adjustment and maternal trauma-reflective functioning. *Frontiers in Psychology*, 10. doi:10.3389/fpsyg.2019.01062.

Dollberg, D. G. & Hanetz-Gamliel, K. (2023). Therapeutic work to enhance parental mentalizing for parents with ACEs to support their children's mental health: A theoretical and clinical review. *Frontiers in Child and Adolescent Psychiatry*, 2. doi:10.3389/frcha.2023.1094206.

Ensink, K., Normandin, L., Plamondon, A., Berthelot, N., & Fonagy, P. (2016). Intergenerational pathways from reflective functioning to infant attachment through parenting. *Canadian Journal of Behavioural Science/Revue Canadienne Des Sciences Du Comportement*, 48 (1), 9–18. doi:10.1037/cbs0000030.

Ensink, K., Normandin, L., Target, M., Fonagy, P., & Berthelot, N. (2015). Mentalization in children and mothers in the context of trauma: An initial study of the validity of the Child Reflective Functioning Scale. *British Journal of Developmental Psychology*, 33203–33217. doi:10.1111/bjdp.12074.

Fisher, J. (2020). *Transforming the living legacy of trauma: A workbook for survivors and therapists*. PESI Publishing & Media.

Fonagy, P. & Allison, E. (2012). What is mentalization? The concept and is foundations in developmental research. In N. Midgley & I. Vrouva (eds), *Minding the child: Mentalization-based interventions with children, young people and their families* (pp. 11–34). Routledge.

Fonagy, P., Campbell, C., Constantinou, M., Higgitt, A., Allison, E., & Luyten, P. (2022). Culture and psychopathology: An attempt at reconsidering the role of social learning. *Development and Psychopathology*, 34 (4), 1205–1220. doi:10.1017/S0954579421000092.

Fonagy, P., Luyten, P., Allison, E., & Campbell, C. (2019). Mentalizing, epistemic trust, and the phenomenology of psychotherapy. *Psychopathology*, 52 (2), 94–103.

Hughes, D. (2016). *Parenting a child who has experienced trauma.* Corambaaf Publishers.

Hutsebaut, J., Nijssens, L., & van Vessem, M. (2023). *The power of mentalizing: An introductory guide on mentalizing, attachment, and epistemic trust for mental health care workers.* Oxford University Press.

Langley-Obaugh, C. L. (2023). We repeat what we don't repair. https://strestllc.com/news/we-repeat-what-we-dont-repair/

Malberg, N., Jurist, E., Bate, J., & Dangerfield, M. (2023). *Working with parents in therapy, a mentalization-based approach.* American Psychological Association.

Meijer, L., Franz, M., Dekovic, M., van Ee, E., Finkenauer, C., Kleber, R., van der Putte, E., & Thomaes, K. (2023). Towards a more comprehensive understanding of PTSD and parenting. *Comprehensive Psychiatry*, 127, article 152423. doi:10.1016/j.comppsych.2023.152423.

Midgley, N., Ensink, K., Lindqvist, K., Malberg, N., & Muller, N. (2017). *Mentalization-based treatment for children: A time-limited approach.* American Psychological Association.

Norbury, J. (2021). *Big Panda & Tiny Dragon.* Penguin Books.

Odgen, P., Minton, K., & Pain, C. (2020). *Trauma en het lichaam: Een sensomotorische benadering van psychotherapie.* Mens.

Slade, A. (2008). Working with parents in child psychotherapy: Engaging the reflective function. In F. N. Busch (ed.), *Mentalization: Theoretical considerations, research findings, and clinical implications* (207–234). Analytic Press.

Weistra, S. R., van Bakel, H. J. A., & Mathijssen, J. J. P. (2024). Adverse childhood experiences in parental history and how they relate to subsequent observed parent–child interaction: A systematic review. *Child & Youth Care Forum*, 54, 755–785. doi:10.1007/s10566-024-09832-6.

Whitefield, C. & Midgley, N. (2015). "And when you were a child?": How therapists working with parents alongside individual child psychotherapy bring the past into their work. *Journal of Child Psychotherapy*, 41 (3), 272–292.

Chapter 11

A parent's perspective on the mentalization-based treatment of a traumatized child

An interview with C. Evans

Emma Morris

C. Evans is the adoptive parent of a 12-year-old girl. She is a single parent. Her daughter is her only child, who experienced very severe abuse while in foster care as a toddler. She only disclosed this to Ms Evans after she was adopted, and it was Ms Evans who reported the abuse to the authorities. The trauma that her daughter experienced impacted across all areas of her development, and still does. The family were referred to a specialist post-adoption support service in the UK and seen for time-limited MBT (Midgley et al., 2017) when her daughter was around six. They attended three rounds of twelve sessions each. Emma Morris worked with Ms Evans, and her daughter was seen by Katherine Mautner (an MBT-trained play therapist and social worker). They came back to therapy again when Ms Evans's daughter was approaching adolescence and had recently started secondary school.

EMMA MORRIS: If I can start with this – what is it like to be a parent of a child who has experienced trauma?

C. EVANS: I had to think about this question a lot because I don't have anything to compare it to. I've never been a parent of a child that hasn't experienced trauma. What I was thinking of to describe it first was just that it's all consuming. That it takes all of your attention and skills and emotions and everything.

But then I thought it's actually very traumatic being the parent of a child who's experienced early trauma. You have to think about the horrible things that have happened to them and they're things that you don't want to think have ever happened to any child, let alone your child. You have to find the words to explain it to them at every age, and you have to keep explaining it in a way that they can understand. Even though you don't really want to, you just want them to know. You just want to say it one time and for them to know that's what happened. But development doesn't work like that, so you keep having to kind of go over it and you have to deal with it.

DOI: 10.4324/9781032713441-16

And then you're also on this incredibly steep learning curve of trying to find out how things work. You're dealing with the complexities of the police and the legal system and trying to make sense of that alongside trying to manage the trauma and just do day-to-day parenting. I think I felt very let down by the agencies that failed her and have continued to fail her. I felt very angry, about the people that hurt her and that this was allowed to happen. And I feel a fierce desire to protect her, but also wanting to kind of burn down everything that caused her to experience trauma.

I'm also thinking about the decisions that I make now, how they'll play out in the future, at some point when I have to explain things to her or when she questions what I did. Will she be happy with the things that I did? Or maybe I'm doing something wrong? I don't know, because I've never been in this situation before and it's something that I don't think many people have experienced. I feel anxious about the future because she's vulnerable to so many things. And what will happen if I'm not here to protect her or fight for her? I feel worried about that.

Then there is just dealing with everyday challenges in the context of trauma – like sleep, food, activities, trying to understand what is going on for her. So that dominates our life, really trying to make sense of what's happening and finding ways to deal with it that are right. I need to educate myself, to live in an entirely new world.

The effects of trauma were something that I didn't know about particularly. I'd had some awareness of it, but not anything extensive, and I certainly didn't know how to manage it. I feel like I've got myself an honorary PhD in trauma now because I've learned so much. I was pushed way beyond the limits of what I felt that I could do. And always trying to separate out what I feel about the situation from what is the right thing to do for her, if that makes sense?

It makes you feel very different from other parents. An example of this is that one of my friends, her little boy was about four, and obviously she loves him very much and is, as all parents are, quite protective of him. But he was playing with a little girl who purposely pinched him, really, really hard. And she was telling me about it. It was hard enough to leave a bruise and, obviously that's upsetting. And she was so furious about it, about this little girl, for doing this. And it just made me think, "Oh my God, if only you knew the kind of stuff." I mean, not to undermine those feelings about her son. But I just felt like, "If only you knew the things that happened to my child that I've had to learn to live with and manage."

I feel like it undermines your belief in ordinary people. Prior to this, I felt like I believed that most people were generally good. And I feel, with this, like I was shown into a house of purely evil people. It took me a long time to really believe what they did. Even though I always believed what my child said, it took me a long time to believe that they had done what she said they did because I kept thinking, "oh, there must be some entirely innocent explanation". It was only when we were in court and they lied and it was a very obvious lie because there were other witnesses there to prove what they had lied about. I think that was the point that I really believed it. It messes with the way that you think about people generally.

EMMA MORRIS: Makes you question your trust and your ability to make judgments about people?

C. EVANS: Yes, because you just don't think about people doing terrible things to young children. It's really unfathomable because every instinct is to protect babies and toddlers and look after them and it's just so hard to get your head around the idea that somebody could hurt them like that and it just makes you really think anybody could do anything to anyone you know.

Now I kind of think that's not true. It's not anybody. It's only certain people, but you don't know who those people are. So I feel less trusting of people. In a way, that's kind of hard to explain. To go from like basically working on the pretext that most people are decent unless you find out something else to go to the other extreme that you think most people are potentially bad. And they have to earn your trust. It's quite hard to live like that.

One more thing – at the time when she made the disclosures, I didn't have parental responsibility. I wasn't privy to all of the information from the child protection medical and all of the court information, and I didn't really understand what had happened at the time. So then later, when she was adopted, then that information was shared with me, but there was no one to really explain it to me and I didn't really understand what it meant. Like the medical things, having to kind of google my way to understand these medical terms. It's just ... I don't know. It's like your world has just exploded. And you have to put it together in a new way. That's just totally different to how you'd expect things to be.

EMMA MORRIS: Is there a sense of loneliness and lack of support around this whole thing? I think you talked about feeling different to other parents.

C. EVANS: Definitely feeling lonely and feeling different to other people. Because it's not something you can just talk about easily, because it makes people very uncomfortable. And people either don't know how to react and want to move on or they have a reaction and then you feel like you have to manage their feelings. You know, if they want to talk to somebody else about it, I wouldn't really want them to be sharing that information and I also have to think about when my daughter's grown up. If she says to me, who knows what happened to her? Do I tell her, like, just the professionals? Or do I tell her, you know, 10 people or 15 people? How's she going to feel about that? Because for everyone to have known something that you haven't really understood yourself – it's just like a lot of things that you have to manage as well as just ordinary parenting, which is hard in itself.

EMMA MORRIS: Absolutely. And can I ask – what do you think is different as a parent of a traumatized child having to support them through school?

C. EVANS: The main challenge would just be about school's understanding of how that trauma plays out in a day-to-day way for her. People kind of have this idea that when things happen to children that they're very young, that they forget about it somehow or that it doesn't have an impact on them. That was a long time ago and now they're fine because they're living with you. People say, "Oh she's lucky, she's lucky to have you". Like, I've got some magic wand.

I don't have anything special. I'm not really equipped for this and she's not OK and I think that's hard for people to understand that she can still be affected by the things that happened to her when she was very young. And my experience in schools has been that they tend to say no, she's doing fine or all children do that, even though they can see that she's not doing fine. I've just found schools really disappointing that you have to send your child to this place every day. And sometimes kind of forcing them to relive their traumatic experiences. And not taking account of her needs.

EMMA MORRIS: Can you think of an example like that?

C. EVANS: In my experience, her school has found it very difficult to understand that her mental health is affected by what happened to her when she was small and that it still has an impact on her now. The things that they're doing to her. The detentions and isolation and punishment. Causing her so much stress that she can't function and it's not helping to improve her behaviour because her behaviour isn't happening because she's naughty, it's happening because she doesn't feel safe.

And throughout her education people have really struggled to understand how she could not be feeling safe because she looks one way, she doesn't look like she's scared. Especially if she's feeling scared, she will act like she's the most confident person in the world and people really find it hard to understand.

EMMA MORRIS: So as a parent, you're left with the job of trying of having to try and make people understand that.

C. EVANS: Yes, as a parent I'm trying to make them understand what things are going to be helpful for her and what things are going to make her be successful. But I think this general feeling in education is that maybe the mother is just being a bit fussy or it's not really happening because we're not seeing her. She's not presenting as scared and she's not presenting as a child that's struggling. It's hard for them to understand. But she's masking her feelings and emotions.

I just wish that schools would listen to the parents more and accept what the parents are telling them rather than dismissing it and thinking that they know better when they can do something else. Since she's been at secondary school, it's just like watching her drown. You know? It's like you can see she keeps going under [crying].

EMMA MORRIS: I'm so sorry. Take a minute.

C. EVANS: You know, if they listen to you, the things that they could do would really help her and make a difference to her, make her be successful and happy. I think that kind of focus on the kind of behavioural systems and punishing and expecting that children can modify their behaviour doesn't help. When they've experienced early trauma and they're really messed up in terms of their relationships with adults, things don't work the way that schools would expect that they would work for typically developing children. It just results in her being punished more and more because she's not able to modify her behaviour to be like someone who doesn't have early childhood trauma.

EMMA MORRIS: They're asking her to do something that she's not capable of doing, and then they're punishing her when she doesn't do it.

C. EVANS: And punishing her for not doing it. And expecting that she'll be able to do it as a result of being punished. Whereas in fact it makes a less likely to be able to do it. Yes.

EMMA MORRIS: OK. We're going to go to thinking now a bit more about therapy. So the first time you came to therapy – oh, my gosh, how old was your child then?

C. EVANS: OK. Yes. She must have been six.

EMMA MORRIS: She was little, so I'm asking you to remember back a long way, but if you can remember what brought you to therapy the first time.

C. EVANS: The first time mainly because she just didn't sleep. And she woke up screaming every night and I thought it was just not sustainable for both of us to be going without sleep. We weren't functioning. I wanted to have some objective kind of measure about how she was coping and the level of attachment that she had to me. We did a story stem assessment initially to look at her attachment. But really, the thing that brought me there really was the lack of sleep and feeling that I was so sleep deprived that I could end up doing something dangerous because I just wasn't getting enough sleep for probably four years by that point.

EMMA MORRIS: So you had some questions in your mind, you wanted to understand her attachment to you a little bit more. But the main thing you wanted to almost get fixed if you like, was the sleep.

C. EVANS: Yes. The sleep was the main thing I wanted to get fixed and I guess I felt like, am I doing attachment right? I didn't know how to measure it or whether it was OK. In my mind I thought that I should be able to make things better by something that I was doing or not doing because I felt like if she had a good attachment to me that I'd be able to calm her. I think that's what I thought, at the time.

EMMA MORRIS: So what did you expect from therapy?

C. EVANS: I expected a magical solution.

EMMA MORRIS: Oh, sorry, that didn't happen for you [both laughing].

C. EVANS: Obviously. I feel cheated. Don't put that in! But seriously, I thought someone else could deliver and that a specialist person who knew about it would be able to do something quite quick, specific. Seems ridiculous now, but I just really felt like if we went to therapy, it would fix it.

I thought it was the right thing to do, but also, I'm probably a bad person because I really did not want to go to therapy week in, week out, which is mad because I've been doing it on and off for like 10 years. I was like, "Oh, I don't want to have to go every week." You know, just wave your magic wand.

EMMA MORRIS: And that's completely understandable. But for you personally what was it you didn't like about the idea of coming every week? Was it the kind of just the inconvenience of it or was it the kind of stigma of it?

C. EVANS: Not the stigma. I don't care about that. It was just like, logistically, it was difficult to get her to go. There were lots of times that she just refused and then we'd have to stop and start again.

EMMA MORRIS: Right, yes.

C. EVANS: I found it really stressful. She has this way, when she doesn't want to do something, of kind of causing a level of chaos which made it quite hard for me to think and follow normal routines. I remember one time we left her school bag on the train and then we had to go all the way back to retrieve it. And I lost my card another time, when I tapped on the tube because I don't know what happened. And then it was logistically difficult, with getting her back to school and then getting into work – I just really wanted to go home and lay down.

EMMA MORRIS: Yes, I was just remembering what you're saying about it being all consuming and then this is another thing on top of something that's all already all-consuming and taking you way beyond your limits.

C. EVANS: Yes, but even when I knew it was the right thing for her, and it was what I wanted for her. It was still difficult to do it all.

EMMA MORRIS: What did you expect before the first meeting? What did you feel?

C. EVANS: I felt really annoyed that it had taken so long because I had to go through the adoption support fund and deal with a social worker. And then it just took a really long time to get an appointment, which wasn't your fault at all. I felt really frustrated from having to deal with so many agencies. And having to jump through so many hoops. I remember when in our first session, [the co-therapist] kind of acknowledged that it had taken a long time for us to get an appointment and I appreciated that even though I knew it wasn't her fault, it was nice for somebody to say that. Just to kind of acknowledge that it had been hard to get there. And I feel like I was a bit suspicious of therapy as well. I could see that my daughter needed it, but I didn't really understand how it works. I think I had this conversation with you quite a lot of times. I don't want it to be like all those cliches about therapy like, you know, the pictures that are what are they called – Rorschach, is it, with the ink blots? Yes, and just lying on the couch and all that kind of stuff. So, I was quite suspicious, but also thinking it was going to help. I mean, I really think there wasn't anything left for us to try really. To fix things.

EMMA MORRIS: You talked earlier on about how being a parent of a traumatized child kind of makes you question your trust in other people. Do you think any of that came into your feeling suspicious of therapy to start off with?

C. EVANS: Yes. I think so. It's quite hard to trust people. If people have said things to me like, oh, you know, make sure she has a good routine and read her story and all that about sleeping I just probably would have head butted them!

EMMA MORRIS: I'm glad I didn't say that then [both laughing].

C. EVANS: I mean, I definitely wouldn't have gone back. I did find it hard to trust the process and the people. But I was always really grateful to you and [my child's therapist] because you never said anything that was like cliched parenting advice. I can't really think of a good example, but always really grateful that neither of you ever said any of the kind of tired parenting cliches that I would have already tried a million times, so I always felt like when I talk to you both, that you got it, you understood it and you weren't being patronizing.

EMMA MORRIS: So what were your first impressions when you first went to therapy?

C. EVANS: The really welcoming and child friendly staff on the reception, they were really lovely and kind. The way the room was set up, there were lots of plants and stuff around and toys and it felt like a space for children. And I didn't feel worried about my daughter doing something to mess things up. I thought that was OK and when other families were waiting there as well, I felt like it was, maybe not friendly but welcoming. I guess it felt like there were other people that were needing support as well. And sometimes, you know, when people had the appointment, always before you, you get to have a little bit of a chat with them. I think the routine was quite important to my daughter as well. To have this routine about going and what happened. I think it was helpful for her as well to see that other children were coming every week.

I felt like I was in a place where I didn't have to worry if they would understand or how much to disclose – I felt like it was safe for me. I always felt that you were both on our side and able to work with us and meet us where we were. Sometimes I did feel a little bit, "Oh, my God, she's being a bit difficult. But I didn't ever feel like the two of you thought that she was being difficult." You probably did. I don't know. I didn't feel judged.

EMMA MORRIS: So what do you think it was like for her coming to therapy?

C. EVANS: She hated it. So I had to create a routine for us, I had to be consistent and it had to be positive. I think she did get better at going and more relaxed about going and it sort of became part of our weekly routine and there were some parts of it that I know she really loved like all the messy stuff and some of the toys and things I know she really liked. And I think she liked it when we all had a session together.

And I think, even though it was difficult, it's good groundwork for her because I feel like she's going to need support throughout her life. Probably. It's not just as I had hoped. One magic person that can fix everything quickly. You know, she's going to need to get support at various stages in her life, I think, and so to have good experience when she's young sets her up to be able to access that when she's older and to know what a good therapy experience is. She'll have like a template of how it would feel if it was good. I feel like just having that relationship was very important to her Even though you were kind of asking her to think about things that she didn't want to think about – that was horrible for her. But to be able to do that somewhere where she felt safe, was really important. I think it was also important that there were two of you.

EMMA MORRIS: How so?

C. EVANS: I think because she was seeing [her therapist] and I was seeing you, it was like we were both participating – it wasn't a case that I would take her and sit outside and wait. I think for us both to do it and then if we had like a joint session, I think she would like those. I think it was important to her that I was doing something as well, that it wasn't just something was wrong with her, you know?

EMMA MORRIS: And you also said she really liked the mess. Do you want to say anything more about that? Do you think that's particularly relevant?

C. EVANS: She did really like the mess. And do you remember she had a little story? Where she had the pink and the blue fluff and the little unicorns?

EMMA MORRIS: Yes.

C. EVANS: Yes. So she really liked that. And making mess with the hand sanitizer and the sand and the paint and all that.

EMMA MORRIS: So the sensory stuff, the touchy feely messy stuff was important for her.

C. EVANS: Yes, the sensory things, and even now.

EMMA MORRIS: OK. And then for you, what was it like for you coming to therapy?

C. EVANS: I feel like it was useful to have space for me to think about things because you're just trying to do all the day-to-day stuff like make this food, make sure the clothes are clean. The house is relatively clean. get her to school, go to work, do all the other activities. But all the time in the back of your head, there's this – not exactly a conversation, but just like thoughts going on in your head about, "Oh, God, there must be a better way of doing this? Maybe it would be better if I did this", or, "Oh, God, just why doesn't she sleep?" Well, you know, like problems with school or friends or whatever. So all of these ideas and thoughts are in your head, but you don't really have anywhere to have a space to bring that to. That was really helpful because otherwise my head was just full of thoughts and worries and ideas and so to have some structure to think about that was helpful because then I could go, "OK, well, I don't know, but I can ask Emma."

To know that there was going to be a space where you could talk about things. I found that really helpful.

EMMA MORRIS: I remember there were points where we thought about you as a person and why you might respond in certain ways and a little bit about your background and your history. Given that you were bringing your child and she was like the "patient", how did it feel for you that I would ask you about things like that sometimes?

C. EVANS: I did find it really useful to have this space to think about what I was doing and how to parent. It was helpful to have someone that I could talk openly with. I liked having the kind of repetition and explanations. Like, how does therapy work? And how does the mind work and how are these memories organized or not organized and why are they always coming out in her sleep. I found that really useful to think about because also at the time I just couldn't read. I know that sounds weird. I've always been like a big reader. And so if I ever didn't know something or didn't understand something, I'd go and find out about it and read something. I think from when she was little I probably went five or six years without reading anything more than Peppa Pig. It's like my brain wasn't working. I couldn't concentrate or read a book. I just couldn't do it. So you know, there was no way I could have sat down and read even though I bought loads of books about trauma and adoption. I did read some of them, but mostly I just couldn't make sense.

EMMA MORRIS: So that psychoeducation part and just going back over that and linking that to help you understand what's going on in the moment that was helpful for you?

C. EVANS: Yes helpful and I think I needed quite a lot of prompting about the mentalization. Because I feel like that wasn't very natural to me to say to her, "Oh, I think you're feeling like this." And even though I was curious about what was going on for her, I wasn't used to being curious out loud. I found that quite hard to get into, that habit of doing that. I found it really helpful and I think it's like one of the things that has actually really worked for her. But it wasn't very natural to me to say those things out loud. You ask people what they're thinking or what they're feeling, but you don't normally say I think you might be feeling blah blah blah.

EMMA MORRIS: You don't. You don't naturally …

C. EVANS: No. And you kind of expect that people will know how they're feeling, don't you? So I found that like quite hard to get my head around, how to do that. That was quite tricky for me. So it was good to have somebody to kind of explain it to me repeatedly. And we needed to practise to do it.

EMMA MORRIS: That's really helpful because as therapists, we're so used to this sort of thing that we can assume that it is a bit more natural because we do it just as part of our day-to-day work.

We often ask parents questions about themselves that don't necessarily relate immediately to the child, but might help us understand why they find certain parts of parenting difficult. With us, I remember there was something about asking for help and there was a point at which we thought a bit about your own childhood and your own experience of being parented, what it means for you to ask for help and what might get in the way. What was that like for you?

C. EVANS: I felt like I could understand why you were asking those questions, because the template that you have for parenting is often based on your own experience of being parented. I don't think I found it particularly uncomfortable. Some of it was painful like the relationship breakdown with my sister and things I found quite painful to think about. But I don't remember feeling that it wasn't relevant or that I didn't see the point of it.

EMMA MORRIS: So, moving on a bit, can we talk some more about how therapy was helpful for your child?

C. EVANS: Just being able to sleep. I can't tell you enough just the difference that makes even though now at times of stress, it's still difficult for her, but just that not waking up and screaming in the middle of the night, that was just so horrendous. Just to know that I can go to sleep and know that I'm not going to get woken up by someone screaming. That was massive. Like I can't explain the hugeness of it. Also, I think dealing with emotions and thinking about emotions for her, being able to name her own emotions, that was important for her.

I don't know if you recall this, but when it was her birthday and the two of you had a little party for her, she made all those confetti and threw it everywhere. It was so lovely for her to have that. It's like part of bringing her life into the therapy. That was a place that by that stage she felt safe enough that she could say: "it's my birthday, I want to have a party".

I don't know really what I'm basing this on, but sometimes I feel like professionals, you're kind of not allowed to see them as humans. Do you know what I mean? Like people have to be professional, which is right and proper. But I always felt like we weren't just seen as patients, we were seen as people, individuals and as a family and I feel like it was important to have that kind of interaction as humans. Does that make sense?

EMMA MORRIS: It makes real sense, and there's something that's not about words to do with that, isn't there? There's something about just a way of being together.

C. EVANS: Exactly. And you know, I think that every week that we came, you always seemed happy to see us like it was never "here they are again, the millionth time" – it was always welcoming. Do you remember, she used to do all sorts of things like hide under the desk or hide somewhere. You know there's always like a bit of a rigmarole starting the sessions, but that kind of playfulness, I think is important for children as well.

EMMA MORRIS: Yes, that playfulness helped her relax a little bit.

C. EVANS: Exactly. And also the other thing I've mentioned a few times was about the routine, was having the same room, I think was quite important to her. All the routine and the structures are really kind of supportive for her, I'd say.

EMMA MORRIS: Do you want to say anything else about how it helped you?

C. EVANS: I think it made me a better parent because I didn't really understand what I was dealing with at the very beginning. I didn't understand how the impact of her early trauma would reverberate throughout the years as she grew.

If somebody had said to me, you could go to therapy or you could just take this tablet. I'll be like, yeah, give me the tablet. But long term, to have the understanding of her and her needs is something I can fall back on if I feel frustrated or annoyed or angry. I know that like I can always take a step back and go, hold on, the reason she still loses her zip card every morning is because she doesn't really want to leave the house. OK, she doesn't want to go out because she doesn't want to leave where she feels safe. And that is easier to manage than just thinking, "Why the hell can't you find your zip card ever?!"

EMMA MORRIS: And then as a parent I imagine if you've got that understanding of her losing her zip card every morning, you get less stressed. And if you're less stressed, you can manage better?

C. EVANS: I don't know. I still find it infuriating, but you can just say to yourself. No, you know, it's because of that, just calm down. Think, "OK, you're not helping anything by reacting like that. That's not going to make it better." You have to think about why. Why is she doing these things? And then once you understand the reason why, then you can maybe try and put something in place or it just makes you a bit more compassionate.

You hear so much about therapeutic parenting. Then actually learning to do it yourself. For me, it was quite unnatural. Because the way that you're brought up and educated – ideas about how children behave and what you should do don't necessarily match. For example, if children are fussy eaters people are quite judgy about that. They'll be like, well, don't make another meal for them. Just give them the food. I remember when she was little, somebody said to me, just give her the meal. And if she doesn't eat it, just don't give her anything else. You think, "Oh, OK." Maybe that is the right thing to do because, you know, I don't want to have a fussy eater that will only eat 12 things, and nine of them are pasta. But you feel like, "OK, maybe I'm doing this parenting thing wrong. I'm a new parent and maybe that is the right thing to do." But then I was like, "What am I doing?" I'm actually abusing her by withholding food.

It's not the right thing to do at all. The things that people say to you don't work with traumatized children. And it's hard to understand that and say, oh, well, actually, no, that's not going to work with my child.

Everybody's saying, "oh, this is what you do for this situation", you know? But it doesn't work. I think that this goes back to me being grateful to the two of you for not saying things like "get a nice sleep routine", because it's so tedious to be told over and over again, "Oh, you just do XYZ" and it just does not work.

EMMA MORRIS: So my question then to you is you've got people telling you to do things that don't feel natural and that don't work, and then you've got me telling you to be curious out loud about your daughters mental states which also doesn't feel natural, and you don't know if it will work straight away or not. What made you stick with that and what made that feel OK over, say, other people's advice to just not give her any more food?

C. EVANS: I felt like it wasn't doing her any harm. A lot of the stuff around sleeping and eating and behaviour is generally a bit punitive and it could be harmful, I think, to children. I could also see that she didn't recognize certain feelings and got things like tiredness, hunger and thirst mixed up. And sometimes she just couldn't tell me what she was feeling, I couldn't make sense of it. I think that's why I kept trying, because I think I kept coming back to you saying, "but I don't know what to do about this". And you kept saying, "remember about the mentalization", and I'll be like, "oh, OK, yeah". I think it took quite a while for me to have that as a strategy that I would reach for first. I think it is the kind of thing that you would do maybe with a 2-year-old like "oh, you're having a tantrum because you're really tired and we're just going to pick you up and give you a drink and tuck you into bed and read you a story. And then you'll have a rest and you'll feel better." But it feels odd to be doing that with a 7-, 8-, and 9-year-olds.

EMMA MORRIS: Anything that you think was unhelpful or less helpful?

C. EVANS: I don't really remember anything that was less helpful or … I don't really remember anything that I thought was not helpful and generally I remember it all being very kind of positive experience.

EMMA MORRIS: Did you feel able to give feedback if I was on the wrong track?

C. EVANS: [Laughing] I was just, like, "no".

EMMA MORRIS: But what was it that allowed you? Do you think that's just because you're kind of a confident, fairly assertive person, or was there anything that I did that helped you be able to say no?

C. EVANS: Probably just because of the length of time that we saw each other. Do you know what I mean? I think probably if I'd come right at the beginning, I might not have said no. But I think after a while, I felt like you both knew us really well and I think generally you were just spot on about things. I can't even think of any specific examples, but I do remember a couple of times saying no, I didn't agree. I think it's just kind of having that open relationship.

EMMA MORRIS: So you've said something about getting to know you and build up a relationship that means that you feel like you can say no. It's helpful for us when parents tell us when we're getting things wrong. The parent could be sitting there thinking that's definitely load of crap and we really want them to be able to tell us when that's the case because it does happen.

C. EVANS: Yes, I think you were quite good at saying, "Does that sound right?", or tell me if that's not right or something like that. I don't think you ever said, "Well, you have to do X, Y and Z." Like you were always checking in. And sometimes I thought, "Oh, I don't know, does that work?" Nobody really knows.

EMMA MORRIS: No, we're all guessing. Did you feel able to talk openly about all your thoughts, feelings, and experiences without worrying about judgement, and if so, what enabled you to do that? And if not, what could I have done differently?

C. EVANS: I definitely didn't feel judged. I think at the very first session I'd said something about how bad things were at night-time. I remember I told you that she was screaming one night I saw that there was a hammer that I'd been putting things up on the wall with and I thought to myself, I should put that away, because if she wakes up screaming, you know, I might go mad and attack her with a hammer. I think you know, quite rightly, they were worried hearing a parent saying things like that, but I didn't mean that I was going to hit her with a hammer, it was just it just crossed my mind that I should put it away. And then I thought to myself, "Oh God, this is really bad." If I'm thinking to myself that I'm going to lose my mind because I'm so sleep deprived, I think I was using that as like an illustration of how bad it was.

EMMA MORRIS: Like how desperate you were feeling. But having just met us, maybe worried that we might judge you for saying something like that, or interpret it the wrong way?

C. EVANS: Obviously as professionals you have to look at the risk, and I remember you asking me whether I was drinking alcohol or stuff, which I didn't because I was so tired I would just fall asleep after one sip. I was just being really upfront about how bad it was. But obviously you have child protection procedures in place and you know you can't have parents going around hurting their children. Yes, I think that was one point that I was like, "Oops, I shouldn't have said that." But I always felt it was better to be entirely open and honest about it because I just thought, what is the point of going if you're not being honest?

EMMA MORRIS: It feels like you were saying from the beginning "I've got nothing to lose. I'm desperate for help. I'm going to tell you everything and let's just hope things get better." For other parents, can you think about things that a practitioner might do to help them to be open and to not feel judged?

C. EVANS: I think being clear about what the sessions are for and what the kind of make-up of it is and what you can and can't keep confidential, what things you can talk about. Being open from the beginning, like if there is something that we're concerned about that obviously we'd have to make a referral because I think that is quite frightening for parents. If they're asking for help and then being judged, I mean, I think that could be, really frightening.

EMMA MORRIS: If you could choose three things to advise every therapist working with traumatized children and parents, what would they be?

C. EVANS: Just, number one, appreciate how much work the parents have done to get to a point that they are coming to therapy because it's not easy to get your child there. Well, it wasn't easy for me to get my child there and it's hard and it's uncomfortable, particularly for the child. And to get to a point where they're coming to therapy, they've probably been through all kinds of difficult experiences and tried all sorts of things, so I think to have that awareness is important. I don't know particularly what therapists think, but it's not like you've just phoned up, made an appointment, "Let's go". Do you know what I mean?

I would recognize that the parents are just ordinary people dealing with extraordinary situations that they maybe don't have the knowledge or the skills to navigate. And you bring your own stuff to the situation, all your past comes into the parenting. I don't know whether you'd agree with this, but I would assume that most people that are bringing their child to therapy are doing absolute the best that they can.

EMMA MORRIS: I would agree with that.

C. EVANS: I think if there's things that you think are wrong about the person or that they're doing something in a way that's not helpful, to always have compassion for people because they're probably doing the best that they can do at that time under those circumstances.

Three things ... I would think for the children being welcoming and having a sense of joy and playfulness. I think that's really important to children, maybe even more so if they've experienced trauma because there's a kind of ordinary, normal childhood things that maybe traumatized children have not always been able to have playful, joyful experiences. I think some of the bits where my daughter made most progress was when she had that good, happy connection with someone. I feel like that was really important for her.

EMMA MORRIS: And are there things that you would advise therapists working with traumatized children and parents not to do? I've already heard you say, "Be really clear, don't give advice. Don't be judgy."

C. EVANS: I would say don't underestimate the complexity of how early trauma plays out in a child's life after the trauma. I think it's so complicated. It's so difficult to work out which bits are trauma and what's something else? You can't, really. And just don't say any of those cliche things about sleeping or eating because we've probably tried all of those things and they didn't work and we did do them right, but they didn't work.

And one more thing. As far as it's possible don't miss sessions and that kind of thing, because especially for my daughter, it was really hard to get her to go and having that consistency in routine was really important to her. I mean, obviously, of course people get sick and have childcare problems and whatever and those things are unavoidable. But where possible to stick to the routine.

EMMA MORRIS: OK, great. And then the last question, are there questions you would like to ask me?

C. EVANS: Oh, any questions? How does therapy work? [both laughing] I don't know. I feel like there's still like something that's a bit of a mystery to me about that. I feel like it would be quite good to have some kind of general information for parents about that, because I feel like I don't know. Do other people ask that?

EMMA MORRIS: I don't think I've ever been asked it so many times as I have by you! But do you know what, it makes me think that I obviously didn't do a great job of explaining it, so that's really helpful for me to think about. I wonder if when you say how does therapy work, you're talking more about the kind of play in the room, like what she did with her therapist?

C. EVANS: I just feel, because she had such a severe trauma and it was so difficult for so many years in terms of her sleep especially, I feel like it's just like a mystery. Like, how come? I don't know. I suppose it's sort of like, I guess, kind of marvelling at the fact that she was so traumatized and then how could that get so much better?

EMMA MORRIS: I don't think it's what happens in the room that makes them better. I think that what happens in the room starts something in them that means when they leave that room, they're a little bit more open to learning, being supported and cared for, and that's where the magic happens.

C. EVANS: A lot of the stuff that she would talk about with me after the therapy – I don't think she would have done that if she didn't go to those sessions. I guess I'm just curious about how it all works and how the brain works and how memories work.

EMMA MORRIS: Next career! You'd be brilliant.

Reference

Midgley, N., Ensink, K., Lindqvist, K., Malberg, N. and Muller, N. (2017). *Mentalization-Based Treatment for Children: A Time-Limited Approach*. American Psychological Association.

Chapter 12

Youth protection services

Working with those who care for traumatized children

Vincent Domon-Archambault and Miguel M. Terradas

Clinical illustration

Joaquim is a 6-year-old boy accommodated at l'Étincelle, a residential unit for boys aged 6 to 12 from a youth protection (YP) rehabilitation centre in Québec, Canada. He joined the unit in an emergency a month ago, following an intervention in his family. Neighbours had contacted YP after witnessing the child's father grabbing him violently by the arm and dragging him to their apartment, yelling. The assessment of the report and associated examinations revealed that the child and his siblings had been subjected to significant physical abuse, psychological violence (e.g. yelling, threats, insults) and neglect in terms of stimulation and supervision. However, the parents did not acknowledge the dangerous situation and refused to cooperate with YP.

On his arrival at l'Étincelle, Joaquim appeared petrified. He spoke very little and obediently followed the childcare workers[1] as they showed him around the unit. The child soon displayed significant difficulties. He refused to be left alone in his room, sometimes shouting and throwing objects if asked to do so. He interacted with other children in a controlling and aggressive manner, for example, trying to take away their toys or forcing them to follow him by pulling their arms. When the childcare workers intervened, Joaquim could suffer major crises. He could attack the other person by biting or spitting at them. If directed to a calming room, the intensity of his crisis escalated and he could end up scratching his face, urinating in his underwear or banging his head against the wall. Marie, Joaquim's designated childcare worker,[2] felt overwhelmed. She told her colleagues she didn't know how to calm down this child, as she couldn't foresee or prevent his outbursts. Joaquim was highly suspicious of her and often felt attacked by the other children and childcare workers. The one-to-one meetings she had with the child did not allow her to access what he was experiencing internally and, therefore, to understand Joaquim well enough to help him better. The child talked very little. Joaquim's arrival also left the other eight children in the group feeling very insecure. A number of them reportedly regressed in terms of functioning, adopting aggressive behaviours themselves or requiring greater proximity to adults. The childcare workers' team was exhausted.

DOI: 10.4324/9781032713441-17

Youth protection in Québec

Unfortunately, Joaquim's story is common in Québec's YP services. Between April 2022 and March 2023, 135,839 reports were processed across the province (Directeurs de la protection de la jeunesse, 2023). These reports have been rising steadily over the last few years. For 42,821 of these youths, the child's development and safety were deemed to be in danger according to the law due to the proven presence or significant risk of parental abandonment, neglect, physical abuse, psychological abuse or sexual assault, or severe behavioural problems. Of these reports, more than 31,000 concerned children aged 12 or under. Nearly 3,000 were placed in rehabilitation centres or group homes. The choice of placement depends on the child's needs and difficulties. These young people, like Joaquim, present challenges too great to be integrated into a foster family. Indeed, most children living in rehabilitation centres or group homes suffer from complex trauma and experience significant developmental, behavioural, and emotional difficulties.

In practical terms, this means that daily childcare workers in the YP services have to deal with children who present several difficulties, including an increased tendency to somatize, act out, and behave aggressively (Domon-Archambault et al., 2019). These young people find it difficult to rely on a relationship with an adult for support and regulation, and this search for closeness may even increase their distress (Bonneville, 2010). As a result, childcare workers find themselves in frequent crisis and aggressive situations. A study by Geoffrion and Ouellet (2013) of 586 YP childcare workers in Québec found that more than half had been the victim of a significant act of physical violence by a youth in the past year. The childcare workers were also subjected to psychological violence several times a week.

Childcare workers often feel powerless and helpless when faced with these actions. This leads to significant challenges in terms of staff retention while putting the adaptability and resilience of those who remain on the job to the test. These organizational issues can lead to an increased amount of aggressive behaviours among children in care, creating a vicious circle from which it is difficult to escape: a child's behaviour increases the risk of resorting to restraint or isolation measures (Geoffrion et al., 2022). It also encourages the use of medication (Desjardins et al., 2010).

In short, it is easy to see that the situation and difficulties experienced by Joaquim, Marie, and the childcare workers' team are common to most YP rehabilitation centres. Childcare workers are in great distress and are looking for clinical support to enhance their understanding of these children's behaviour, give meaning to their aggressive gestures, better deal with, and adapt to them (Lamothe et al., 2021).

Mentalization-based interventions in youth protection: helping childcare workers help children

In response to these various needs and observations, we have developed an approach based on mentalization for childcare workers working in YP rehabilitation centres. In light of the systematic clinical observations we carried out in YP and the empirical work on the subject, it seemed clear that the acting-outs, somatization and crises of these children could be explained, at least in part, by their mentalizing difficulties (Yang & Huang, 2024; Domon-Archambault et al., 2019). Research carried out among children in YP care in Québec confirmed our hypotheses (Dubé et al., 2019; Fournier et al., 2019).

This approach had several potential advantages in the context of YP rehabilitation centres. Firstly, as mentalization is a developmental achievement, mentalization-based intervention (MBI) can be applied to all children, regardless of the severity or diversity of their clinical profiles and diagnoses. Secondly, work in a school context demonstrated the effectiveness of an approach based on mentalization in reducing children's acting out and aggression (Twemlow et al., 2005). Thirdly, children in rehabilitation centres evolve in a context that is similar to a family environment, which gives rise to common emotional and affective issues comparable to those they might experience within their family. These are natural conditions for the development of mentalizing capacity (MC) – and for potential mentalizing breakdowns. The same applies to the attachment relationship that children develop with their childcare workers, an essential dimension in the development of mentalization. Fourthly, teams like Marie's are usually trained in attachment theory, which has several links with mentalization. Fifthly, we wanted to develop an approach that could be easily integrated into childcare workers' day-to-day activities with the children in their care. Finally, the approach does not require the acquisition of complex skills or knowledge; rather, it relies on a capacity that childcare workers already possess. It simply asks for them to observe themselves and to improve their interventions based on their observations. The aim is to develop what we call the *mentalization reflex* in childcare workers: how can I use what I'm doing with the child, in the here and now, to help them to mentalize more?

Development of a training manual

The approach was developed and tested in its early stages (Domon-Archambault & Terradas, 2015a, 2015b). An intervention manual was created and refined over time and through experience. The manual (Domon-Archambault et al., 2023) comprises four sections in its current format. The first section explains the context of the interventions and their objectives. We stress the need to establish specific goals to guide the interventions undertaken with the child and evaluate the child's progress. The second section covers theoretical concepts relating to mentalization, the characteristics of the parent-child relationship necessary for its development, the dimensions of mentalization, and prementalizing modes. It also addresses the consequences of complex trauma on the development of the MC. The third section is devoted to the clinical assessment of children's MC. Childcare workers learn to assess the child's mentalization resources and difficulties by observing the child's behaviour, relationships with other children and childcare workers, and the characteristics of the child's stories, play, drawings, and other artistic productions. The childcare worker also learns to assess the child's predominant prementalizing mode. This information will guide the interventions offered to the child.

In the manual, we also describe the reactions and emotions that the child might elicit in the childcare worker depending on the child's predominant prementalizing mode(s). Clinical examples enable childcare workers to identify moments when their own MC may diminish in response to the child's behaviour. The childcare worker too could eventually lose their MC and function in a prementalizing mode. The fourth and final section is devoted to MBI. In the first part, we look at the childcare worker's posture and attitudes, which encourage the deployment of their own MC and that of the child, as well as the main parameters of the approach. In the second part, we discuss specific interventions based on the child's predominant prementalizing modes. In the third part, we present other interventions that can promote the development of a child's MC. Finally, in the fourth section, we look at interventions to develop the child's imaginary world and ability to pretend, skills closely linked to MC (Target and Fonagy, 1996). Throughout the manual, we pay particular attention to providing information in layperson's terms and use several examples to illustrate the concepts (Domon-Archambault et al., 2023)

Training l'Étincelle child care workers

Since its creation, in addition to the work carried out as part of the research, the approach has mainly been offered to teams expressing an interest in it. Marie's team approached us with a request for training. The training of the l'Étincelle team was spread over five months. The childcare workers and the department head first participated in five three-hour training sessions. Four two-hour intervision meetings followed these sessions. The training and meetings were held bimonthly. The total duration of the training is designed to help make the most of the intervention. Activities between the meetings enable the childcare workers to keep the mentalization approach in mind. The continuity of the approach is guaranteed by the participation of the department head and by the occasional presence at team case discussions of a clinical advisor previously trained in MBI.

Part 1: training meetings

We began the first training meeting by explaining to the seven childcare workers in Marie's team and their department head the rationale behind the development of the approach. This crucial icebreaker validates and accepts the powerlessness and suffering experienced by those involved in care daily. Raoul, a childcare worker with twenty years of experience, spoke about the increasing clinical burden of children in care. Janna, a young childcare worker, said that she hardly expected to experience almost daily assaults when she chose this profession. Talking about these experiences and corroborating them with data from the literature helped lay the foundations for an exchange tinged with humility, openness, and non-judgment. This is a critical step in ensuring that the training takes place in a friendly and participative way. We then looked at some of the challenges associated with working with children who have experienced complex trauma:

1 incomplete development, characterized by disharmony in cognitive, emotional, and social functioning;
2 epistemic mistrust, reflected in hypervigilance towards childcare workers as new attachment figures; which has repercussions on their
3 difficulty in managing interpersonal distance in relationships with childcare workers and other children;
4 idealization of abusive parents;
5 emotional and behavioural disorganization manifested in frequent and intense outbursts of anger;
6 a regressive return to bodily sensations (e.g. swinging like an autistic child) and manipulation (e.g. compulsive masturbation) in the event of distress;
7 poor imaginative capacity, which translates into difficulties in the ability to play and understand metaphors; and
8 psychological functioning in survival mode, with primitive defences that are often ineffective.

By using humorous or salient scenes and images involving, for example, well-known political figures, we get childcare workers to engage their MC without their knowledge. Ingue, for instance, shared her hypotheses on what Hillary Clinton's forced smile in one of the photos might be hiding. This exercise then enables childcare workers to intuitively co-construct a collaborative definition of mentalization, supplemented by theoretical content. For example, one team member might talk about reflecting on their experience, while another might talk about metacognition. Depending on their backgrounds and knowledge, each team member contributes their grain of salt and seeks to make the definition their own. The commitment of l'Étincelle's childcare workers was strong at the time, and many questions emerged about the links that could be made with other concepts, such as empathy or the theory of mind. The adaptations made possible by mentalization were described in detail, as were the effects of deficiencies in MC.

During the second meeting, we discussed the definition of mentalization and its development. Emphasis was placed on the elements conducive to healthy development in the child's attachment relationship with the parent, mainly through the prism of the mirroring function (Winnicott, 1963). The concepts of sensitivity, holding, empathy, congruence, contingency, differentiation, and respect for the child's cycles of engagement and disengagement are particularly well supported (Fonagy & Target, 1996; Target & Fonagy, 1996). The members of Marie's team welcomed this section with interest, making many links with their training in attachment. Eva also noted that the elements of the mirroring function are still relevant in how childcare workers respond to children's needs. Prementalizing modes were then described in detail, using examples from normal development. The team was silent during this part. Our experience in training has taught us that these concepts are complex and require much time for childcare workers to integrate and assimilate. However, these elements are central to the approach since a large part of it is devoted to assessing the child's predominant prementalizing mode and using adapted intervention strategies.

The third meeting dealt with the impact of complex traumas on the mirroring function and mentalization, as well as identifying the predominant prementalizing mode in children. This section explains various manifestations of the teleological, psychic equivalence and pretend modes observed in children in rehabilitation centres (see Table 12.1). This provoked numerous reactions from the childcare workers, who made connections with their daily lives. Marco pointed out, for example, how Isaac, a 7-year-old boy in the unit, displayed several facets of the teleological mode, unable to pretend while playing and to grasp the childcare workers' jokes. Isabelle noted that Luis, aged 8, displayed many manifestations of the psychic equivalence mode since he perceived hostility towards him in several perfectly harmless interventions. The meeting ended with presenting three clinical cases in which the childcare workers were asked to work together to identify clues that might suggest difficulties in the parent's mirroring function and the child's predominant prementalizing mode.

When they arrived at the fourth meeting, the childcare workers shared the results of several discussions about prementalizing modes and the children in their unit. Raoul noted that his view of the children in the unit had changed because he had a better understanding of how their mentalization difficulties could explain behaviours that were previously difficult to understand. He gave the example of Luis, who, when angry, accuses Raoul of provoking him when Raoul asks empathetically what Luis is feeling inside. Raoul observed that he had a better grasp of the fact that Luis was not intentionally trying to make him angry but was rather struggling to understand that his mental representations differed from the other person's. A quiz presenting brief case

Table 12.1 Manifestations of prementalizing modes observed in children who have experienced difficulties in a YP setting.

Prementalizing mode	Behaviour, attitudes and relationship patterns	Characteristics of narratives, play, drawings and other artistic productions
Teleological mode	Focused on concrete, observable aspects of experience. Body-centred affective regulation (e.g. somatic reactions and complaints, acting out, aggression, overexcitement). Angry outbursts when overwhelmed by emotions. Difficulty in obtaining an integrated view of internal experience, as this is not necessarily represented. Describe their experience in terms of a succession of somatic states or observable behaviours that are more or less related to each other. Tendency to refuse dialogue when not feeling well. Difficulty in understanding how to relate and interpreting non-verbal signals suggesting mental states in others.	Poor narrative and few references to mental states. Literal understanding of what others say. Difficulty in understanding humour and metaphors. Poor imagination: difficulty in developing stories, choosing a game and explaining the game to the childcare worker, inability to imagine that an object could represent something else. Focused on physical games involving motor release. Difficulty in pretending and symbolizing. Concrete interpretation of artistic productions. Concrete use of different means of expression.
Psychic equivalence mode	Difficulty distinguishing one's own thoughts from those of others: tendency to think that the child care worker knows or remembers everything there is to know about them or, conversely, to assume what the child care worker thinks without verifying it. Tendency to project what they think onto others. Affective regulation centred on controlling others or, conversely, on total harmonization with the thoughts of others. Hypotheses put forward by the childcare worker are understood as real or, conversely, what the child is experiencing is experienced as real. Reliving the trauma as if it were happening in the moment rather than as a memory.	Difficulty in pretending, because what is represented in the game seems too real and authentic. Difficulty in creating stories or drawings that allow them to identify with imaginary characters. Rigidity: objects can only represent what they are or the function assigned to them socially. Not feeling the need to explain games, drawings and other artistic productions to the childcare worker. Assuming that the childcare worker knows what they want to do, without having to explain it. Tendency to reproduce well-known games (often video games) in a rigid manner. Deviation from the scenario or the familiar characters in these games is not allowed. Equivalence between what is represented and what they feel: can be overwhelmed by the use of symbolization media, because the internal states called upon are experienced as too real.

Prementalizing mode	Behaviour, attitudes and relationship patterns	Characteristics of narratives, play, drawings and other artistic productions
Pretend mode	Understanding of self, others and the world around them is disconnected from what is going on around them and devoid of authentic emotions. Impression given of being a small adult or trying to reverse roles with the childcare worker. Use of avoidance, intellectualization, rationalization and projective identification to regulate emotions and behaviour. May experience feelings of emptiness and confusion, and feel that they have difficulty understanding themselves. May behave in a *false self*, i.e. according to what they think others expect of them. May react very neutrally to stressful situations. Often takes the childcare worker's words literally, without necessarily understanding them.	Preference in talking over acting. Interest in current events gives the impression of pseudo-maturity. Rigid speech that does not correspond to that of a child of the same age. May also engage in apparently mentalizing speech, but have difficulty relating what they say to their inner experience and to what is happening in their immediate environment. Impression given that they talk for the sake of talking, that their speech is rather empty, that they take refuge in an imaginary world or that they resort to dissociation to manage their difficulties. Proposed scenarios often represent idealized situations. Confrontation with elements linked to their psychological or environmental reality tends to inhibit their imagination and, consequently, interrupt their play. Graphic production: little connection between the drawing and what they say about it. Artistic production: little emotion in connection with their work.

Source: inspired by Allen (2008), Fonagy et al. (2004), Gergely (2003), Verfaille (2016) and Verheugt-Pleter et al. (2008).

examples was used to consolidate the childcare workers' ability to identify the clinical manifestations of prementalizing modes. As with mentalization, the emphasis was on the childcare workers' reflective process rather than on giving the right answer. Ingue noted that the terms associated with mentalization, in particular prementalizing modes, were complex to integrate. A decision tree outlining the main questions they may ask themselves to identify the child's predominant prementalizing mode(s) was given to the childcare workers (see Figure 12.1).

The rest of the meeting was devoted to MBI adapted to the childcare workers' interventions. The general idea was to encourage them to slightly modify their daily interventions, often simply by making implicit natural processes more explicit and encouraging them to use their mentalization processes to help the children develop their MC. First, there was the question of how to adapt intervention objectives based on targets associated with mentalization. Eva found the approach interesting because she was revising an intervention plan for Hugo, the child in her care. She stated that she appreciated the fact that she could have a specific target, such as working on a particular mental state, or a more general target, such as increasing the frequency of the child's mentalization of others.

Next, the childcare worker's posture when using MBI was presented. Isabelle noted that the not-knowing stance differed from her usual position as a childcare worker, who seeks to identify as quickly as possible what is happening to a child by offering a definite response to make the child feel secure. We made links with the tendency of some children to repeat exactly what their childcare workers tell them, without this having anything to do with their internal experience in the present moment (staying in the pretend mode). A child who recently had a conflict with a peer may, for example, cite a distant family visit as the source of their emotions in the here and now since this hypothesis is often raised in connection with their behaviour. The childcare workers said they appreciated the approach's spontaneity, "common sense", and naturalness. They said they were open to referring to themselves when talking about mental states, noting that they did not necessarily spontaneously resort to this type of intervention.

As a next step, the general principles of the intervention approach were described. These include security, active collaboration, empathy, the zone of proximal development and scaffolding, play, and the reduction of non-mentalizing interventions. The team was very receptive to the elements discussed in this section, again comparing them with how they currently operate. Marie noted that thought should be given to ensuring the emotional security of childcare workers to support their MC. The idea that the mentalization of the adult promotes the mentalization of the child thus took on its whole meaning for the childcare workers. Ingue suggested reflective spaces during the children's break times and a dedicated discussion time at team meetings. The childcare workers also found it refreshing that the approach encouraged them

IDENTIFYING PRE-MENTALIZING MODES: WHAT QUESTIONS SHOULD CHILDCARE WORKERS ASK THEMSELVES ?

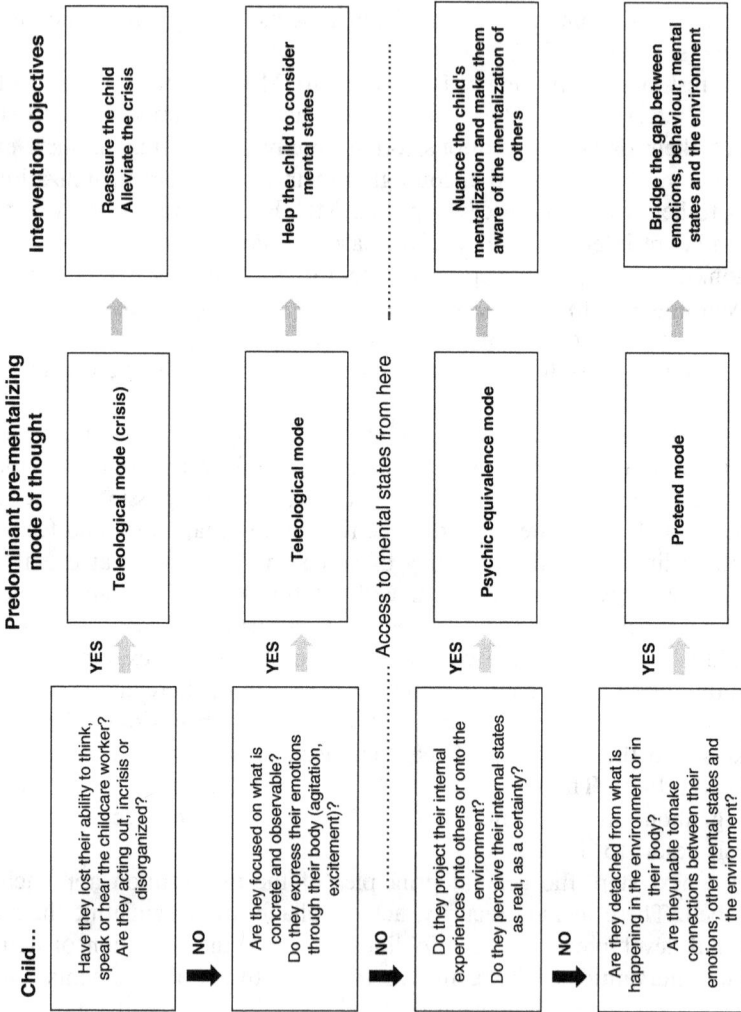

Child...

Predominant pre-mentalizing mode of thought

Intervention objectives

Have they lost their ability to think, speak or hear the childcare worker? Are they acting out, incrisis or disorganized?

— YES → Teleological mode (crisis) → Reassure the child / Alleviate the crisis

NO ↓

Are they focused on what is concrete and observable? Do they express their emotions through their body (agitation, excitement)?

— YES → Teleological mode → Help the child to consider mental states

NO ↓

.... Access to mental states from here

Do they project their internal experiences onto others or onto the environment? Do they perceive their internal states as real, as a certainty?

— YES → Psychic equivalence mode → Nuance the child's mentalization and make them aware of the mentalization of others

NO ↓

Are they detached from what is happening in the environment or in their body? Are theyunable tomake connections between their emotions, other mental states and the environment?

— YES → Pretend mode → Bridge the gap between emotions, behaviour, mental states and the environment

Figure 12.1 Identification of the child's predominant prementalizing mode.

to intervene in positive or play moments to stimulate the children's mentalization. Finally, the team seemed receptive to focusing on the mentalization process rather than the precise identification of a mental state. Although this may seem paradoxical at first glance, it takes the pressure off them to work with hypotheses in mind when dealing with children who are sometimes difficult to understand.

The last part of this meeting dealt with specific interventions based on the child's predominant prementalizing mode. First, intervention in the context of behavioural disorganization was described. This section is essential in the context of increased restraint and seclusion measures in rehabilitation centres. Some of the basics of brain function, in particular the response to acute stress in children who have experienced trauma, are presented to set the stage for the proposed strategies. Suggestions were given on intervening before, during, and after such a crisis. Particular emphasis was placed on the impact of unintentionally making children relive traumatizing events, in particular by leaving them alone in a room when they are having a crisis. The childcare workers found this section very relevant in supporting parents as they prepare to send children home and in managing crises in the unit.

Specific interventions were then proposed based on a child's predominant prementalizing mode (see Table 12.2). These consider the limitations and abilities associated with each mode while proposing ways to help the child develop the skills needed to pursue the development of their MC. Eva said she appreciated that several proposed interventions were relatively concrete and easy to implement. We feel that this balance between general principles and practical measures is crucial. Finally, some additional interventions were described. These are concrete methods aimed at supporting the mentalization process more generally and can be used with both children and their parents. Thinking aloud or using techniques such as the "mentalizing hand" (Allen & Fonagy, 2012) or the film[3] (Allen, 2008) were examples presented. The end of this session dealt with interventions to stimulate a child's ability to engage in pretend play. Concrete ways of supporting pretend play, storytelling and imagination were then presented. Marco said that he found this part very interesting. He explained that play is often used during support meetings with children in follow-up care. However, the childcare workers noted that they knew little about how to use it to promote the development of the child's MC. The meeting ended with a review of the clinical cases discussed. This time, childcare workers were asked to think about MBI that could be deployed with children and their parents.

The fifth training session aimed to consolidate what had been learned in the previous sessions. It also discussed teamwork based on mentalization, inspired by the "thinking together" model Bevington and Fuggle (2012) proposed for hard-to-reach individuals. We began this section by saying that it was highly likely that the different members of the team had various ways of understanding the difficulties of the children with whom they worked.

Table 12.2 Objectives and examples of actions to be taken with children depending on their predominant prementalizing mode.

Predominant mode	Objectives of the interventions	Examples
Teleological mode	Encouraging children to consider mental states (e.g. thoughts, emotions, intentions) in their understanding of themselves and others. Helping the child to gradually focus less on what is concrete and observable and more on what is not (e.g. the emotions underlying a behaviour). Supporting the decoding of behaviours and non-verbal signals (e.g. gestures, easy expressions) indicating the presence of mental states in oneself and others.	During pretend play, the childcare worker can mime more and exaggerate the facial expressions of the emotions of the characters portrayed in the game so that the child has access to them.
Psychic equivalence mode	Promoting the distinction between the child's internal world (their mental representations), the world of others (self-other differentiation) and their environment (self-non-self differentiation). Encouraging the mentalization of others and helping children to nuance their self-representations in order to decentralize them from their egocentric perspective.	When a child reports a confrontation with a friend, the childcare worker can provide alternative explanations for the friend's behaviour.
Pretend mode	Establishing links between the child's mental states, behaviours and physical sensations and what in the immediate reality could have given rise to them. Helping children to anchor themselves in reality by reconnecting them to their own somatic expressions and to the mental states and behaviours of the people around them.	When the child's speech becomes distanced from their internal experience (e.g. the emotions underlying their behaviour) and from what is happening in their immediate environment (e.g. a confrontation with their parent), jointly identify the starting point and the mental states that produce this distancing.

Sources: inspired by Allen (2008) and Verheugt-Pleiter et al. (2008)

Similarly, we emphasized that the same child could elicit discordant reactions from different childcare workers. Marie pointed out the discrepancies between a designated childcare worker's understanding of the child with whom they are working and that of the other team members. She added that the childcare worker often has access to information (e.g. emotions discussed during a one-to-one meeting) that other workers do not. Marco pointed out that the childcare worker's reactions to the child they are working with are "less objective", as they are often more attached to the child. Raoul added two interesting points. First, he pointed out to his colleagues that the childcare workers take their work so seriously that sometimes they give the impression of talking about the child in their care as if they were a member of their family. In his opinion, this shows that childcare workers are "really" attached to the children. Occasionally, they may forget that it is crucial to maintain optimum relational distance between themselves and the child. Raoul said that the childcare worker assigned to the child is not always the best person to intervene with them. In his opinion, whenever possible, the team should work together to determine the most appropriate person to intervene with a child, depending on the nature of the intervention to be carried out. We suggest that the team see disagreements as common and normal, not as a sign that someone is doing something wrong or does not understand the child's problems. In this approach, we take the time to reflect on the differences and similarities of opinion between the team members while considering the internal experience of the childcare workers and not placing the blame on anyone. This transforms the pitfalls of differences of opinion into opportunities to gain an enriched understanding of the child's difficulties (Bevington & Fuggle, 2012).

The final point addressed in this meeting concerned the childcare worker's own mentalization. We emphasized that the childcare worker's MC, like any other person, can be put to the test, eroded, and even completely inhibited in certain circumstances (Bateman and Fonagy, 2013). We then addressed the idea that childcare workers can operate in a prementalizing mode when faced with situations that generate significant distress. We then gave some examples. Childcare workers operate more teleologically when they draw conclusions about a child solely based on observable behaviour without considering mental states that might explain the child's behaviour. They operate in psychic equivalence mode when they assert that they know what a child is thinking and do not question their assumptions. Finally, childcare workers who apply the same interventions to all children with whom they work without adapting them are likely to be operating in pretend mode. We then invited the l'Étincelle childcare workers to add their own examples of prementalizing functioning in childcare workers.

Part 2: intervision meetings

We believe it is almost impossible to appropriate this intervention approach without a subsequent intervision process, a type of peer supervision guided by the trainers. Indeed, the use of clinical assessment and interventions based on mentalization is much more effective when it can be tested directly with childcare workers who reflect on the youth in their unit. In what follows, we describe one of the early intervisions conducted by the team at l'Étincelle.

At this first intervision meeting, Marie offered to talk about Joaquim. We first invited her to present the following elements: the reason for his placement in YP, the child's life and family history, and his behaviour towards the other children and the childcare workers in the unit. Next, we asked Marie to present a situation where she would like to do things differently and use MBI. Marie discussed the need to deal with tantrums differently, as her current method was ineffective. Although she seems to manage to remain calm during Joaquim's tantrums, she insists that he obey a series of rules (e.g. no throwing objects, go to his room to calm down), which provokes more agitation and opposition from the child. We encouraged Marie to reflect on the mental states this situation was generating for her and Joaquim. She said she felt frustrated and powerless. She also felt embarrassed by the possibility that her colleagues would think she is not a good childcare worker. Marie cannot stop thinking that Joaquim is angry with her for not giving him more time and that he is throwing these tantrums to provoke her. We then invited the other team members to share their hypotheses about Joaquim's mental states.

This was followed by a clinical assessment of the child's psychological functioning as part of the intervision. The team concluded that Joaquim functions more in a teleological mode. Raoul brought up the reasons endangering the child's development to support this hypothesis. Living in a context of neglect, it is highly likely that Joaquim did not receive much feedback from his parents to help him better understand his feelings (Fonagy et al., 2004). In addition, his father's violence could have caused the child to withdraw defensively from the mental world to avoid thinking that his father had malicious intentions towards him (Allen, 2008). Janna identified behaviours in Joaquim that could be associated with the teleological mode: difficulty regulating his emotions and his self- and hetero-aggressive behaviours. Marie recounted that during a conversation with another child after a fight at school, Joaquim had trouble identifying his feelings towards his classmate. She no longer offered him free play periods, as he was rather concrete and could not put himself in the character's shoes. Marco highlighted an important point: when Joaquim became suspicious of the childcare workers, he seemed to project his hostility onto others, which reminded him of the psychic equivalence mode.

At the end of the intervision, the team decided to focus initially on managing Joaquim's tantrums. The aim of the intervention during the crisis would not be to get him to mentalize more; it would be to make him feel more secure. We are talking about the notion of *survival of the object* by Winnicott (1963) to introduce the idea that crisis management represents a major challenge for most childcare workers. Marie would try to speak only a little, make simple requests, and not respond to the child's provocative words and behaviour. Knowledge of how the brain works suggests that the child may experience the childcare worker's verbalizations as excessive stimuli that clutter the child's psychological system (Allen, 2008). Interventions to promote the development of the child's MC can be carried out systematically *after* each crisis. Marie would first try to re-establish contact with Joaquim in a non-verbal way by showing him her reassuring presence (e.g. she could sit close to him without saying anything). She would then ask him to go through the sequence of events that led to the state of uncontrollable stress he experienced; the aim being to jointly develop hypotheses that could explain his feelings and behaviours.

During this type of intervention, it is essential to remain attentive to the child's reactions, as some children may show a kind of emotional reactivation when the crisis is mentioned verbally. In this case, explaining that the crisis was over and that reflecting on it would not lead to further disorganization might be appropriate. Finally, it would be important to identify the impact of Joaquim's aggressive gestures on the other children and the childcare workers during the crisis without making him feel guilty. This intervention would aim to help Joaquim understand the mental states underlying the behaviour of others towards him after the crisis. For example, another child might not want to play with Joaquim for fear of being attacked by him. It was agreed that the other childcare workers would intervene similarly when Marie was absent and remain attentive to take over when a crisis was prolonged. In a second phase, Marie would begin to provide interventions to support the development of Joaquim's imagination and pretending skills. The team thought that it would probably be necessary for Marie to introduce an imaginary world to facilitate the emergence of pretend play in the child. She could also dramatize and exaggerate the expression of affects through play to give explicit access to the mental states underlying the behaviour of the various characters. Similarly, Marie could simulate sensations and exaggerate the characters' reactions in the pretend play. The intervision group hoped that these interventions would teach Joaquim to play with reality, an essential element of MC.

Our experience is that intervision is most helpful when careful consideration is given to the conditions that encourage learning in this context. First, we invite childcare workers to adopt a mentalizing posture. It involves colleagues adhering to the same attitudes (e.g. adopting a not-knowing stance) and parameters (e.g. allowing oneself to play with ideas) that set MBI boundaries with children in care. The aim is to create a safe space where the childcare worker presenting situations with the child in their care feels sufficiently confident to mentalize in the presence of their colleagues. Second, we emphasize the importance of validating, normalizing, and holding the emotions, powerlessness, and momentary losses of MC of the consulting person. Third, we encourage childcare workers to name difficult emotions that are not always expressed openly (e.g. anger, shame, and negative emotions aroused by the child). We explain that this process will help us to understand the situation entirely. Fourth, it is essential to emphasize the childcare worker's benevolent intentions behind unsuccessful attempts to intervene. Fifth, we discuss the importance of supporting the development of strategies to maintain the MC of the person presenting the situation if there are instances of overload. For example, the childcare worker could ask a colleague to take over in a crisis when they become angry at a child's oppositional behaviour. Sixth, we encourage childcare workers to focus on concrete examples when thinking about intervention. It is like recreating the problem in the here and now. This makes it possible to use interventions equivalent to those used in film or photography to explore the situation in an intervision context. Finally, we propose questioning and supporting mentalization about the child, the self and the relationship to give meaning to what appears to be expressed in the behaviours of the child and childcare worker. In this way, the team can confront the childcare worker's presuppositions and support the development of alternative hypotheses.

Conclusion

The l'Étincelle childcare workers said they found the training enjoyable and useful. They noted that the theoretical content was relevant to their work, the clinical cases aligned with their experience in the field, and the approach was easily integrated into their current way of doing things. The way the training was delivered and the atmosphere within it also appealed to the childcare workers. However, the team members find it difficult to change the posture they usually assume to work with children's externalized behaviours and modify the intervention techniques they use to make more room for MBI.

Humility, respect and humour are at the heart of how we present our approach. We also give numerous examples from our clinical experience to complement the material. We also think with teams about how they will maintain the approach once the training has ended. This often involves someone from the team taking responsibility for on-going work within the approach. In addition to the department head and the clinical advisor, Marie volunteered to be the *guardian* of the approach going forward. She will, therefore, ensure that the approach is kept alive at l'Étincelle, notably by continuing group discussions similar to the intervisions. The main challenge is to make the approach sustainable. Children in protective care put the childcare workers' MC to the test daily, and staff turnover remains high.

Like all work with children who have experienced trauma, there are challenges. To date, the training has only been given to YP teams who had expressed an interest both in Québec and France. Several efforts have been made to evaluate the impact of training on how childcare workers intervene and, on the MC, and internalized and externalized behaviours of children in care. However, staff turnover is a significant obstacle to research. Although modest, the results indicate that the training supports acquiring new intervention knowledge and encourages more explicit use of childcare workers' MC (Rigaud-Larose et al., in press). We also observed a significant reduction in depressive symptoms, social problems, somatic symptoms, attentional disorders and internalizing disorders in children aged 6 to 12 in care following the training of childcare workers (Domon-Archambault et al., 2019).

Regarding the next steps, one of the most important YPC in Quebec recently asked us to train a group of 40 childcare workers working in different rehabilitation units and accepted to integrate a research protocol to the training. We hope to continue collecting research data to prove the benefits of MBI in the context of child protection.

Notes

1 In Quebec, childcare workers' educational background is quite varied. Technical programmes (special education, for example), bachelor degrees (psychology or sexology, for example), or master's degrees (criminology or psychoeducation, for example) can all give access to the profession.
2 The designated childcare worker is the person in charge of the child's specific file. For example, they arrange appointments and care, hold individual meetings with the child and help to draw up the child's care plan.
3 Following Allen (2008), we suggest to the child describing the situation that led to the failure of his MC as if it were a movie. It is therefore possible to go back, move forward, or change the scene; to revisit the situation and better understand what made his MC to fall down.

References

Allen, J. G. (2008). *Coping with trauma: Hope through understanding*, 2nd edition. American Psychiatry Publishing.

Allen, J. G. & Fonagy, P. (2012). Individual techniques of the basic model. In A. W. Bateman & P. Fonagy (eds), *Handbook of mentalizing in mental health practice* (pp. 67–80). American Psychiatry Publishing.

Allen, J. G., Fonagy, P., & Bateman, A. W. (2008). *Mentalizing in clinical practice*. American Psychiatric Publishing.

Bateman, A. & Fonagy, P. (2013). Mentalization-based treatment. *Psychoanalytic Inquiry*, 33 (6), 595–613. doi:10.1080/07351690.2013.835170.

Bevington, D. & Fuggle, P. (2012) Supporting and enhancing mentalization in community outreach teams working with hard-to-reach youth: The AMBIT approach. In Midgley, N., & Vrouva, I. (Eds.), *Minding the child: Mentalization-Based Interventions with children, young people and their families*. Routledge.

Bonneville, E. (2010). Effets des traumatismes relationnels précoces chez l'enfant. *La psychiatrie de l'enfant*, 53 (1), 31–70.

Desjardins, J., Lafortune, D., & Cyr, F. (2010). La pharmacothérapie dans les centres de rééducation: portrait des enfants placés qui reçoivent des services médicaux. *La psychiatrie de l'enfant*, 53, 285–312. doi:10.3917/psye.531.0285.

Directeurs de la protection de la jeunesse. (2023). *Bilan des directeurs de la protection de la jeunesse/Directeurs provinciaux 2022: En équilibre vers l'avenir*. Production des directeurs de la protection de la jeunesse/directeurs provinciaux.

Domon-Archambault, V. & Terradas, M. M. (2015a). Les interventions fondées sur la notion de mentalisation auprès des enfants en situation d'hébergement. *Revue québécoise de psychologie*, 36 (2), 229–262.

Domon-Archambault, V. & Terradas, M. M. (2015b). Efficacité d'une formation fondée sur la notion de mentalisation auprès des intervenants en centre jeunesse: étude pilote. *Revue québécoise de psychologie*, 36 (3), 183–208.

Domon-Archambault, V., Terradas, M. M., & Drieu, D. (2023). *Mentaliser en contexte de protection de l'enfance: guide à l'intention des éducateurs*, Université de Sherbrooke.

Domon-Archambault, V., Terradas, M. M., Drieu, D., De Fleurian, A., Achim, J., Poulain, S., & Gerrar-Oulidi, J. (2019). Mentalization-based training program for child-care workers in residential settings. *Journal of Child and Adolescent Trauma*, 13, 239–248.

Domon-Archambault, V., Terradas, M. M., Drieu, D., & Mikic, N. (2020). Mentalization-based interventions in child psychiatry and Youth Protection Services II: A model founded on the child's prementalizing mode of psychic functioning. *Journal of Infant, Child and Adolescent Psychotherapy*, 19 (2), 321–334.

Dubé, G., Terradas, M. M., Didier, O., Guillemette, R. & Achim, J. (2019). Empathie, mentalisation et comportements extériorisés chez les enfants d'âge scolaire hébergés en centre jeunesse. *Revue de psychoéducation*, 48 (2), 347–371.

Fonagy, P., Gergely, G., Jurist, E. L., & Target, M. (2004). *Affect regulation, mentalization, and the development of the self.* Other Press.

Fonagy, P. & Target, M. (1996). Playing with reality: I. Theory of mind and the normal development of psychic reality. *The International Journal of Psycho-Analysis*, 77 (2), 217–233.

Fournier, S., Terradas, M. M. & Guillemette, R. (2019). Traumas relationnels précoces, représentations d'attachement et mentalisation d'enfants en contexte de protection de la jeunesse: mise à jour des connaissances et application au contexte de protection de la jeunesse. *La psychiatrie de l'enfant*, 62 (2), 433–453.

Geoffrion, S., Lamothe, J., Drolet, C., Dufour, S. & Couvrette, A. (2022) Exploring reasons motivating the use of restraint and seclusion by residential workers in residential treatment centers: A qualitative analysis of official reports. *Residential Treatment for Children & Youth*, 39 (4), 416–436. doi:10.1080/0886571X.2021.1973940.

Geoffrion, S. & Ouellet, F. (2013). Quand la réadaptation blesse: Éducateurs victimes de violence. *Criminologie*, 46 (2), 263–289.

Gergely, G. (2003). The development of teleological versus mentalizing observational learning strategies in infancy. *Bulletin of the Menninger Clinic*, 67, 113–131.

Lamothe, J., Geoffrion, S., Couvrette, A. & Guay, S. (2021) Supervisor support and emotional labor in the context of client aggression. *Children and Youth Services Review*, 121, doi:10.1016/j.childyouth.2021.106105.

Rigaud-Larose, F., Terradas, M. M., Machado da Silva, T., Parr, V., & Domon-Archambault, V. (in press). Effets d'une formation sur la mentalisation sur la capacité des éducateurs à intégrer cette approche en protection de l'enfance (Effects of a mentalizing training on the child workers' capacity to integrate this approach in Youth Protection). *Revue québécoise de psychologie*.

Target, M. & Fonagy, P. (1996). Playing with reality: II. The development of psychic reality from a theoretical perspective. *The International Journal of Psycho-Analysis*, 77 (3), 459–479.

Twemlow, S. W., Fonagy, P., & Sacco, F. C. (2005). A developmental approach to mentalizing communities: I. A model for social change. *Bulletin of the Menninger Clinic*, 69 (4), 265–281. doi:10.1521/bumc.2005.69.4.265.

Verfaille, M. (2016). *Mentalizing in arts therapies.* Karnac Books.

Verheugt-Pleiter, A. J. E., Zevalkink, J., & Schmeets, M. G. J. (2008). *Mentalizing in child therapy: Guidelines for clinical practitioners.* Karnac Books.

Winnicott, D. W. (1963). The theory of parent and infant relationships. In P. Buckley (Ed.), *Essential papers on object relations* (71–101). New York University Press.

Yang, L., & Huang, M. (2024). Childhood maltreatment and mentalizing capacity: A meta-analysis. *Child Abuse & Neglect,* 149. doi:10.1016/j.chiabu.2023.106623.

Chapter 13

The Reflective Fostering Programme

A psychoeducational mentalizing group for foster and kinship carers

Sheila Redfern and Nick Midgley

Introduction

> *Connor, 11 years old, lives with his grandmother because his parents cannot take care of him anymore. He can be very aggressive: shouting, hitting out at his grandmother, Janice. Janice sends him to his room, telling him to stop being so naughty all the time. She feels helpless in managing his outburst, and guilty towards her own daughter, feeling she has done things wrong in her upbringing.*

As of March 2023, there were just under 84,000 young people in care in the UK, of which 65% were removed from the care of their parents because of risk of abuse or neglect, with a further 13% removed because of inadequate parenting (UK Government, 2023). The largest proportion of these children (68%) live with a foster carer, which in some cases may be an extended family member (known as kinship or connected carers). Given that many of these children have experienced trauma following maltreatment in their early lives, it is unsurprising that this group of children have much higher rates of mental health difficulties than their peers. For example, rates of depression are over twice as high, behaviour problems are nine times higher, posttraumatic stress disorder is 12 times higher (McGuire et al., 2022). This constellation of mental health problems often includes a chronic difficulty in establishing trusting relationships, within the foster family or with peers or people in the social environment. This lack of trust in relationships can place foster placements at risk, and placement breakdown is common, with children often moving placements many times (McGuire et al., 2024).

Foster carers in the UK are generally offered opportunities to participate in trainings, including ones aimed at helping them understand how to parent a foster child, deal with challenging behaviours, or understand safeguarding. However, these programmes do not always attend to the experiences and feelings of foster carers in the relationships they have with their fostered young people. Reflective fostering is a model of parent–child mentalizing that was originally devised in the UK for birth parents (Cooper & Redfern, 2016) and then adapted for foster and kinship carers as the Reflective Fostering Programme (Redfern et al., 2018). The development of the approach drew on

DOI: 10.4324/9781032713441-18

the first author's experience of living in a multi-cultural, urban environment (London), and working for over thirty years with families with children who have entered into care, so that the local authority (divided by regions in the UK) becomes the "corporate parent". To date, the programme has been evaluated in two pilot studies, which provide initial evidence that the programme is effective in reducing carer stress and improving the emotional and behavioural well-being of children in care (Midgley et al., 2019, 2021a), and is currently being evaluated in a UK-wide randomized clinical trial, involving local authorities and independent fostering agencies from various regions of the UK (Midgley et al., 2021b).

This chapter sets out the process of one reflective fostering group which was delivered as part of the on-going clinical trial. The chapter pays particular attention to the way trauma impacts the relationships that the carers have with the children in their care, as well as the carers' own capacity to mentalize. The chapter will also set out how these challenges to mentalizing appear in the group meetings; and how weekly supervision was used to help keep the whole group's mentalizing capacity "on track".

The Reflective Fostering Programme

The Reflective Fostering Programme focuses on the practical application of a set of tools for foster carers to use on themselves and on the children in their care as well as the foster family as a whole. The programme consists of ten three-hour sessions delivered by two trained facilitators (one a social work professional, the other a foster carer) to a group of eight to ten carers over a period of four to six months. Originally developed to be delivered in person, it was also adapted for online delivery in response to the Covid-19 lockdown (Redfern et al., 2023). Throughout the programme, psycho-educational discussions, games, exercises, and work sheets are used to support and enhance foster carers' capacity for mentalizing both self and other, with the expectation that this will in turn help to reduce foster carer stress and improve the carer's sense of parental efficacy. The aim of applying the programme in foster care is to support the delivery of high-quality foster care and ameliorate some of the mediating effects of early adversity on children's development – namely their experiences of unsafe relationships and difficulties in understanding other's perspectives and the more nuanced aspects of relationships.

Self-mentalizing plays a key role in the Reflective Fostering Programme, with an understanding that the capacity to self-mentalize is likely to be challenged more severely in the face of caring for children who have experienced developmental trauma. This can often impact on the way the child engages with adults, which in turn unbalances the foster carers' ability to regulate themselves and their capacity to mentalize. The Reflective Fostering Programme therefore emphasizes the importance of tuning into the carer's state of mind, aiming to reduce situations where foster carers are left feeling inadequate at and questioning of their ability to parent in ways that meet the young person's needs. The programme has been developed as a way to improve foster carers' sense of competence and confidence in understanding themselves and their foster child, enhancing their mentalizing capacity, with the ultimate aim to improve foster children's relationships with their carers and, as a consequence, promote placement stability and the outcomes for children in care.

Throughout the 10-week Reflective Fostering Programme, each session introduces a different theme, and a set of specific tools runs through the entire programme:

a   the Professional APP (with APP standing for: attention, perspective-taking, providing empathy: in other words, the mentalizing stance of a supporting professional);
b   the Carer Map (the foster carer's state of mind and capacity to mentalize themselves and others); and
c   the Carer APP (the foster carer's stance in relation to mentalizing their child).

A tool referred to as the "emotional thermometer" is also used to help foster carers bring the level of their emotional arousal into their awareness, and then manage this in order to get into a more reflective, mentalizing range (more details about the programme itself can be found in Redfern et al., 2018).

Meeting a reflective fostering group

The group that we will focus on in this chapter consisted of carers from two local authorities in different parts of the UK. As with the majority of the groups that were part of the clinical trial, it was held online, with carers joining a Teams call remotely from their homes. The group was facilitated by Rickie (a foster carer with substantial experience of longer term and emergency placements) and Mary (a social worker), neither of whom had any prior experience of running groups or of delivering a mentalization-based intervention. As well as having different professional backgrounds, the facilitators were from different cultures: Rickie is white British, while Mary is black British (with Jamaican heritage). As part of delivering the programme for the first time, the facilitators attended a three-day (online) training about the Reflective Fostering Programme, run by the programme developers at Anna Freud; and – once they started to run a group – attended a weekly consultation meeting with an experienced mentalization-based practitioner. The training focuses on two main aspects of delivering the group: (i) modelling mentalizing to the foster carers in the delivery of the materials for each session, and (ii) modelling differences/different minds and perspectives by reflecting on the group process. This is a significant task for inexperienced (and some experienced) group facilitators as they are required to both notice the process in the group and to deliver psychoeducation materials. For this particular group, the consultant from Anna Freud's team was Beth, who offered weekly hour-long consultation meetings to the two facilitators to help them develop their skills and increase model fidelity as the programme progressed.

The group itself comprised six foster carers, with one connected (kinship) carer member. Connected carers are usually family members who, sometimes following care proceedings, have taken on the care of a family member's child. Kinship carers face unique challenges; not only in being related to the child's parent, but in being unsupported both financially and organizationally, compared with foster carers. In this group, the connected carer, Janice, was grandmother to her daughter's 11-year old son, Connor. In Janice's case, the issues relating to developmental trauma take on a greater significance as she carried a great deal of guilt about her own parenting of her daughter, who neglected to meet the needs of 11-year-old Connor. At the start of the group, Janice wanted to learn how to manage Connor's behaviour as she felt he was beyond her control at times. Frequently, carers come to the group because they want to be able to change their child's behaviour, and it is explained early on that an effective way to support change in behaviour is to help the child develop better emotion regulation, which can come about through mentalizing the child. The goals of the group programme are centred around this principle of learning to mentalize the self and other in order to bring about greater emotion regulation in both foster carer (or kinship carer in Janice's case) and in the child in their care.

The other five carers in the group were also female and ranged in ages from 49 to 67. Typically, foster carers tend to be in this age-range and may have their own children who are often older when they decide to foster. In this group the five foster carers and one connected carer were all female and came from diverse backgrounds and experiences in their fostering journeys. Two members of the group, Sam and Keisha, were relatively new to fostering and had been in role for less than two years. Another foster carer, Precious, had been fostering for 15 years and was particularly experienced in caring for adolescents. Precious was the most experienced member of the group, but also felt somewhat ambivalent about the group, and it was noted that, as the only black foster carer in the group, she felt in a minority. Her attendance in the group was sporadic. Precious was looking after a young person who was separated from his family in Afghanistan, and she spoke often about trying to meet the needs of a young man who had a different religious background to her own (he was Muslim and Precious was Christian). The other two members of the group were 67-year-old foster carer Alison and 55-year-old carer Nat. Alison experienced a significant loss of her sister in week three of the group. This had a huge impact on her ability to mentalize herself and it was particularly difficult for her in session 4 (on trauma) of the programme, where the focus is on support networks – her sister was her main support.

Introducing mentalizing to the group

When running a group for the first time, newly-trained facilitators are likely to face a range of challenges. Rickie and Mary, this group's facilitators, came to their consultation after the first session with lots of doubts. As part of the consultation process, the facilitators shared some short clips of the first session, focusing especially on a moment that had gone well, and a moment that had been challenging for them. Beth, the group's consultant, noted that Rickie and Mary were trying very hard with the model, but there were a few obstacles in the way. The sound quality on Teams was poor, and the facilitators seemed to have difficulty in sticking to the model and not falling back on ways of doing things which they were familiar with, even if these did not really fit with a mentalizing stance. In this consultation session, Beth noted that the facilitators were initially anxious about their ability to communicate the programme's meaning, due to their lack of experience. However, she also felt that the two facilitators were extremely open and curious about the group members and this stance of not-knowing, allowed them to model a level of uncertainty which increased the sense of trust in them from the foster carers. They were particularly adept at promoting curiosity and modelling the basic mentalizing stance, but Beth needed to bring them back to the core principles of mentalizing, and support them in developing confidence in running the group. The facilitators were challenged by being asked to hold on to multiple roles when delivering the programme: delivering the psychoeducation material, noticing the group processes and dynamics as well as the group's changing capacity to mentalize themselves, each other and the children in their care.

The first session of the programme begins with an introduction to the concept of "mentalizing". Beth had noticed with other groups that it can take up to session four to five for new facilitators to become comfortable with using the "mentalizing" word. So Beth tried to help the facilitators to use their own language and find a way of describing mentalizing that felt acceptable to the group, as in the first meeting one or two group members expressed their dislike of the word. Alison said that she felt more comfortable talking about being able to be "reflective" rather than "mentalize" and, particularly in relation to their foster child's trauma, she preferred to speak about understanding their "back story".

Over time, the group found its own language to speak about mentalizing, and the challenges to mentalizing that are part of being a foster carer. In week four the group watched a clip from the film *Removed*. It was difficult for the group to watch because the clip shows a foster carer misunderstanding why her foster child is distressed by the dress she has bought for her. The film illustrates that the dress is triggering of her early trauma as the child recalls her mother having her dress torn in a particularly violent argument with her abusive partner. The group members spoke about the way that it's often extremely difficult to understand their children's behaviour, because they don't know details of their early history. However, Rickie and Mary encouraged them just to remain open and curious about the meaning of their children's behaviour and encouraged them to let go of the need to find an explanation or go to an instant fix (i.e. to resist falling into the non-mentalizing modes).

Foster carer Nat was extremely helpful to the group and the facilitators at particular points during the course of the group as she was a naturally good mentalizer and had done some similar training before. It was interesting to note how the other foster carers in the group trusted her experience. They found it helpful when she acknowledged that she often didn't know what to do, but tried to always listen and understand what her children were trying to communicate with their behaviour. Because she was an experienced carer, it impressed the group particularly that she was able to adopt this non-expert stance. The group process can be very powerful in this regard; members of the group are learning how to mentalize from other foster carers as much as they are learning from the facilitators of the programme.

The Carer Map and mentalizing the self

The Reflective Fostering Programme makes explicit to foster carers how their own state of mind can be highly influential on their child's emotional state, and that a greater calibration of these emotions in the carer–child relationship leads to a greater connection between them. Carers with insecure and/or unresolved attachment histories will probably have difficulties in their mentalizing and be more likely to be triggered negatively by their foster child's attachment needs and behaviours (Howe, 2005). This can in turn reactivate the childhood anxieties, traumas, and defences of these foster carers. Unfortunately, this prevents them from being able to successfully attune to their foster child and challenges their sensitivity. It is central to the work that carers are supported to become more aware of how their own experiences contribute to their role; however, some foster carers may find this aspect of the approach difficult. Having simple examples of how past experiences can impact both positively and negatively on parenting also helps normalize this process. Supporting foster carers to reflect on their place in their own birth families, their current circumstances (such as newness to the role) and their current state of mind (e.g. worry for their future finances) are all helpful to developing self-mentalizing, which helps foster carers become more regulated in their interactions with their foster children.

In the second session of the programme, carers are introduced to the idea of the Carer Map, which helps them to reflect on what they bring from their own histories to the current situation. Foster carers themselves may come into the role with their own difficulties and complex experiences of being parented; these in turn, in the face of traumatic presentations, can make the parenting role extremely difficult. Sam, who was a relatively new foster carer, disclosed in session two, that she had been forced to take on a carer role for her younger siblings in her own family as a relatively young child, as both her parents were quite neglectful of her needs and preoccupied with their own lives and difficulties. The effect of these difficulties sometimes interfered with Sam's ability to be present and to think and respond in a reflective manner with her foster child, rather than with her projections, distortions, and judgements of her foster child's behaviours.

Janice was an experienced parent and relatively recent connected carer. When she became a connected carer to her grandson, Connor (her daughter's son) she was faced with the additional difficulty of her own sense of guilt about her daughter's neglect of her son, due in part to her own issues with substance misuse. In the early part of the programme, Janice remained relatively quiet in the group, finding it particularly hard to understand the importance of self-mentalizing as she had come to the group to try to find out new strategies for managing Connor's oppositional behaviour. She expressed her doubt that reflecting on her own role could be helpful to Connor, and said she found the Still Face video in session two, where carers watch a video of a parent responding to a baby without showing any emotions in her face, particularly guilt-inducing as it reminded her of her own difficulty parenting her daughter when she was little. Janice was in the unique position in the group as the only member who was fostering one of her own family. Struggling to manage her grandson's behaviour, Janice would often respond to his aggressive challenges by sending him to his room and telling him to stop being so naughty all the time. Connor would respond by hitting out at Janice and was left with his feelings of shame unresolved, alone in his room, and he would frequently trash his room in these situations.

As the group progressed, other members spoke of their difficulty managing their emotional temperature around their foster children and Janice came to see that she wasn't alone in losing her mentalizing capacity, as the group would frequently become very highly aroused as they talked about the children in their care. It was often a tough task for the group facilitators trying to help the group to notice they were becoming too "hot" to mentalize. The group were validated by the facilitators as they named that the group had gone into a non-mentalizing state when they talked about their children's challenging behaviour; while Janice started to notice that she was in high state of arousal when Connor challenged her, because she felt guilty about her own daughter's neglect of his needs, and her own part in "failing" (in her eyes) to give her daughter the parenting skills she needed. When her arousal was lower, she was able to see that Connor's lashing out at her was his need for control over a situation where he did not have the emotional language to say how he felt and saw his grandmother as being harsh and critical of him (he often misread her face as threatening when she was feeling stressed).

After Janice had reflected on her own Carer MAP and the important influences on her current state of mind, she started to be curious and attentive to Connor's frame of mind when he came home from school, where he had few friends. She started to give him more rather than less attention after school to show him that she was interested in him and in spending time with him. The next time he got angry with her, instead of sending him away to his room, Janice asked him if he could try to calm down and suggested that after he felt calm they could cook the evening meal together. Over time, Connor did this and felt understood and calmer in himself over the mealtime.

Impact of the child's trauma on foster carers

Throughout the programme, but specifically from session four onwards (where the focus is on understanding the impact of trauma), the foster carers started to think about their foster children's difficulties with mentalizing, often arising from being raised by a parent whose mind may have been extremely hard to understand, and where abuse and neglect was often ongoing. Children who have experienced maltreatment may have learned to inhibit their mentalizing function, or may not have developed the capacity to mentalize due to the trauma they experienced to their attachment system (Allen, 2006). Activities in the group, and shared experiences of parenting, helped the foster carers start to see the children in their care in a different light.

One example of a group activity involved asking the carers in the group to draw a Child Map for their children, including their past (to the extent that they knew about it) and current influences. This exercise in mapping out their child's history and current life helped carers in the group get in touch with some of the experiences of their children. This was a difficult exercise for many, particularly Janice as she reflected on the things that had happened in Connor's early life when he lived with his mother. Likewise, Precious came to see that her foster children were not always able to put their feelings and experiences into language; instead, her children had become defiant. Another carer, Keisha, said her foster child had done the opposite, in not being defiant or speaking to her, but instead shutting down and remaining very quiet, which caused her to reflect on what she might feel she could and couldn't talk about.

Through Keisha increasing her understanding of the impact of early trauma (via psychoeducation and group exercises) and her increasing ability to mentalize her foster child, she saw that this was not a deliberate, conscious, effort to defy or ignore her, but rather was the way her foster child had learned to adapt to a parent whose mind was impossible to understand. With this realization came an increased feeling of empathy for her foster children, and a deep sense of sadness often permeated the group discussions about these early experiences, sometimes with elements of anger against the birth parent. This was especially difficult for Janice, with her relationship with her daughter (Connor's mum) at the forefront of her mind. Janice found it difficult to express this inside the group at first, and she asked to speak to the facilitators outside of the group, to first talk about her discomfort in the group as a Kinship carer, and then to think about her own role and how she could bring this into the group. With the support of the two facilitators, she found her voice and her sense of security increased in the group.

The process by which mentalizing the child increases in the group is multi-faceted. One way is by simply being exposed to the thoughts, feelings and experiences of the other carers in the group. By being exposed to multiple perspectives, the foster carers are able to consider an alternative perspective to their own. Another way is through problem-solving exercises such as one where they are given a vignette of a foster child who storms off to his room and are asked to generate ideas about what is going on for him. The emphasis in the group-based activities is on practising the techniques of reflective fostering and applying these by exploring incidents that have occurred at home in the session with the group. The group were encouraged to not focus solely on the external behaviour of their child, but to also keep a focus on the child as an individual with their own mind, and to understand that they often do things for reasons that are linked to how they are thinking or feeling – that there is an inside story. Ricki and Mary sensitively supported the foster carers to respond to that inside story of thoughts and feelings, rather than just reacting to the behaviour.

Many of the carers in the group told stories about how the children's difficulties continued to place great demands on them as carers. The facilitators (and other group members) provided considerable empathy and validation for these struggles, but also encouraged the carers to try to maintain a non-judgmental, non-expert and empathic attitude towards the children in their care. It was notable that one of the more experienced foster carers in the group, Nicky, struggled in facing her foster child's challenging behaviours. Over time, Nicky increasingly reflected on how her own early trauma had affected her parenting and mentalizing capacity. Reflecting on the importance of mentalizing herself, Nicky said:

> In the group, we do lots of work on where the child's at and how they feel ... the side I didn't really do much on before was including myself in it. I wouldn't think about myself in a situation where I was trying to sort out an issue that was going on with a child I was looking after. I wouldn't stop to think, "How does this make me feel? Am I reacting the right way? Is this going to work out?"

By using the Carer Map to work out her own reactions to her foster child and how difficult it often felt to mentalize during particularly challenging interactions, Nicky learned how to step back and make time to think about how these interactions made her feel, and where these feelings were coming from.

Several carers commented that the psychoeducation session around trauma was particularly helpful to their understanding of the impact of their child's early trauma and subsequent behaviour on their own capacity to stay in the "warm" mentalizing range on the emotional thermometer (i.e. to stay within the zone of tolerance). The psychoeducation in this session covers information about developmental and relational trauma; the perceptual bias that can result from having experiences of early trauma and the impact of trauma on a child's relationships, development and behaviour. In discussions that may arise from this psychoeducation, the group model particularly attends to the foster carers' needs in relation to emotion regulation difficulties. Janice faced extreme challenges in her relationship with her grandson and Precious with her teenager foster children which raised their level of arousal, thus compromising their capacity to mentalize. One of the consequences of this rise in emotional "temperature" is a high level of arousal being brought into the group itself. Consequently, the emotional temperature of the two facilitators and their own capacity to mentalize themselves and the foster carers in their group became even more important.

The relationship between the two facilitators

In the way the reflective programme is delivered, the relationship between the two facilitators serves as a model for mentalizing others. Rickie and Mary modelled their different perspectives and experiences of fostering (from a social work and a foster carer's perspective) in a way that gave permission to the women in the group to explore their differences and similarities with one another. In the consultation meetings, Beth noticed that Rickie had a slightly better conceptual grasp of the model than Mary, while Mary was better able to bring her own experiences to the discussions and share her own struggles as a carer in an open and non-defensive way. Beth encouraged them to move a bit more towards each other, while not minimizing their different experiences.

Rickie and Mary thought there was quite a particular quality to running the group online, that meant people don't always have the commitment to fully participating; they noted that sometimes foster carers in the group might be sending a text message or an email or two, but the facilitators were then able to have a group conversation about including this in their ground rules. By having two minds in each session, the balance between commenting on the group process, and delivering the group programme, is easier to manage. It also serves another purpose in further modelling the balance between action and reflection which is integral to the programme and is illustrated through the use of the "two hands" approach to fostering (Hughes, 2006), i.e. the balance between mentalizing the child on the one "hand" and responding to behaviour or setting expectations and boundaries on the other.

In her consultation sessions, Beth felt that the facilitators were showing a good level of curiosity in others, but this could be developed even further, and that doing so could enable the group participants to bring more of their own experiences. She introduced a tool called the Professional APP, which could be used to help the facilitators regulate their own and the foster carers' arousal in these moments of high affect. The Professional APP, which stands for attention, perspective taking and providing empathy, is the facilitators' go-to tool in working with this model. Within the 10-week Reflective Fostering Programme, the facilitators are encouraged to model the stance for the foster carers in their group and use this tool to help them maintain an awareness and control over their own state of mind in relation to the work and the relationship with the carers. The facilitators would increasingly make reference to their own state of mind in the group, for example Rickie sometimes noted that she lost her capacity to mentalize when the technology went wrong and she couldn't make her connection work.

In session six of the programme ('Responding to problematic behaviour in a reflective way'), the group became very animated and went to the high (hot) end of the emotional thermometer during a difficult discussion about how to respond when a foster child tells their foster carer that she hates them or rejects something that the foster carer has spent a long time and care preparing. As the group's emotional temperature increased, the group came out of the "warmer", mentalizing range they had previously been in during a discussion about types of parenting. They started to talk about the importance of rules and boundaries and talk of "showing them who's boss" started to dominate the conversation as the foster carers increasingly lost their capacity to mentalize the child's experience. Activating their professional APP enabled the facilitators to first empathize with the foster carers' feelings of being rejected by their foster children, and then to be curious about what felt so difficult for them about this. One foster carer spoke of feeling her role was constantly under scrutiny and judgement and so when her foster child rejected her, this further compounded her feeling of low value. This conversation enabled the group to start to restore their mentalizing capacity and over time the facilitators, still drawing on the professional APP, started to offer their own different perspectives about times when a child seems to be rejecting what their foster carer is offering, even when it comes from a loving place. By the end of this group activity, the foster carers in the group were more regulated and able to start a process of mentalizing about the traumatic experiences their children had often had in their birth families which had left them struggling to regulate themselves in relationships and also confused about their foster carers' intentions towards them.

Going "beyond" behavioural solutions

Throughout the course of the group, carers often spoke about very difficult situations where they felt pressured to come up with a quick response to a challenging situation. Often in the work either a foster carer or a facilitator will look quickly for behavioural solutions, a response to a situation that will stop it happening or change a child's behaviour. It was notable that Keisha, who was relatively new to the role of fostering, wanted a list of strategies for dealing with the challenging behaviours that can be the result of early trauma.

But reflective fostering requires a degree of discipline on the part of the facilitators to resist the urge to respond directly in this way, as the work resides in thinking through, in relational terms, the states of minds relating to specific situations, wherein often relational solutions can be considered.

On occasions, Keisha persisted in asking for solutions; the facilitators found that a useful technique in response was to try to connect with the thoughts and feelings that may have been underlying Keisha's insistence, and to help her mentalize herself in this moment of high pressure:

> Can I just stop and think with you about something? I am trying to imagine what it's like for you at the moment. I know you are a relatively new carer and the prospect of caring for a child with a history of trauma and challenging behaviour might feel really overwhelming. I'm trying to imagine how it is for you looking after Billy, where nothing seems to be stopping this behaviour. What is that like for you?

Through this kind of approach, Keisha could begin to communicate frustration and a sense of disempowerment, or a sense of incompetence, which is important to discuss and understand as these feelings can be detrimental to forming a more positive and connected relationship. Once Keisha felt understood and had these feelings validated, the emotional temperature began to come down, and she was able to think more freely about what Billy's behaviour indicated about his state of mind, and how she could respond to that, and not just the behaviour. She began to notice, for example, that Billy's behaviour was often most challenging when he felt that he didn't have any choice about what to do, so she began to think of playful ways in which she could offer him options, and he could select which one he preferred. This way she was able to ensure he did what was needed, but without making him feel "trapped". Although this was a behavioural solution, she was only able to come up with it once she'd been able to regulate her emotional arousal, become more curious about the meaning of Billy's behaviour, and come up with a response that responded to that meaning, and not just the behaviour itself.

As this group of carers progressed through the programme, it was poignant to see the sense of community and mutual developing within a relatively short period of time. Groups allow the co-existence of multiple minds, experiences and perspectives and give people exposure to entirely different ways of seeing themselves and their foster children (or grandchildren) which is non-judgmental and empathic. The group continued to meet on a WhatsApp group after the programme finished and still meet to this day, sharing their daily experiences and noticing (in a non-judgmental way) their frequent lapses in their mentalizing. The group support gives them a space to self-regulate and regain their mentalizing with the aid of others in the group. It serves as a constant reminder that trauma in a child's history has a powerful influence over a carer's capacity to retain their own mentalizing capacity and, through implementing the Reflective Fostering tools, it helps foster carers to mentalize themselves before responding to their foster child, which has a profound effect on the stability of the relationship.

Conclusion

For many children in care – including the ones in the group described here – the environment of their early years may have been characterized by a lack of the type of contingent, responsive, and sensitive care essential for accurately reflecting back their emotional states. This sensitive responding is essential to helping a child manage stress as they learn to self-regulate. If instead there is severe ongoing stress, this can alter the structural development of the brain and in turn affect its neural networks and biochemistry (Perry & Hambrick, 2008). Such stressful experiences have a significant detrimental impact on the child's ability to manage extremes of arousal and to regulate their emotions when faced with such arousal.

Some interventions in foster care settings focus primarily on children's behaviours and offering "parenting strategies". While there is a need to focus on problem behaviours, this might not always address the actual difficulties in the relationship between the child and the carers and ignores the importance of the different mental states underlying the problem behaviour. The Reflective Fostering Programme offers a highly collaborative approach aimed at promoting the quality of foster family relationships, supporting effective and sensitive parenting, and breaking unhelpful patterns of relating. The progamme has been developed as a way to improve carers' sense of competence and confidence in understanding themselves and their foster child, with the ultimate aim to improve foster children's relationships with their carers and, as a consequence, promote placement stability and improve outcomes for children in care. The model is strongly based on the premise that foster carers' sense of competence and epistemic trust will be greatly enhanced by completing this programme with other carers, who may have experiences and perspectives that are at times shared, and at times quite different. It is strengthened by the co-facilitation model, bringing together a social care professional and a foster carer, which participants identified as a particular important element of the model, as it helped foster a sense of epistemic trust (Midgley et al., 2021a). The programme views carers themselves as the main agents of change and is based on a view that the children in care should not necessarily be seen as having mental health problems, but more as having a need for consistent and reliable care. Furthermore, by training foster carers in the facilitation of these groups and increasing opportunities for role development of the members of the group, it aims to reduce the stigma attached to fostering, instilling a sense of value and capacity to have the most important impact on the lives and outcomes of children in care. As one foster carer said of her role, "It's the most important thing I've done with my life."

References

Allen, J. G. (2006). Mentalizing in practice. In J. G. Allen & P. Fonagy (eds), *The handbook of mentalization-based treatment* (pp. 3–30). John Wiley & Sons.

Cooper, A. & Redfern, S. (2016) *Reflective parenting: A guide to understanding what's going on in your child's mind.* Routledge.

Howe, D. (2005). *Child abuse and neglect: Attachment, development and intervention.* Palgrave Macmillan Publishers.

Hughes, D. (2006). *Building the bonds of attachment: Awakening love in deeply troubled children.* Jason Aronson Publishers.

McGuire, D., May, K., McCormack, D., & Fosker, T. A. (2024). Systematic review of the impact of placement instability on emotional and behavioural outcomes among children in foster care. *Journal of Child and Adolescent Trauma*, 17, 641–655.

McGuire, R., Halligan, S., Meiser-Stedman, R., Durbin, L., & Hiller, R. M. (2022) Differences in the diagnosis and treatment decisions for children in care compared to their peers: An experimental study on post-traumatic stress disorder. *British Journal of Clinical Psychology*, 61 (4), 1075–1088. doi:10.1111/bjc.12379.

Midgley, N., Cirasola, A., Austerberry, C., Ranzato, E., West, G., Martin, P., Redfern, S., Cotmore, R., & Park, T. (2019). Supporting foster carers to provide reflective caregiving: a preliminary feasibility and pilot evaluation of the Reflective Fostering Programme. *Developmental Child Welfare*, 1 (1), 42–63. doi:10.1177/2516103218817550.

Midgley, N., Sprecher, E., Cirasola, A., Redfern, S., Pursch, B., Smith, C., Douglas, S., & Martin, P. (2021a). The Reflective Fostering Programme: further evaluation of the intervention when co-delivered by social work professionals and foster carers. *Journal of Children's Services*, 16 (2), 159–174. doi:10.1108/JCS-11-2020-0074.

Midgley, N., et al. (2021b). The Reflective Fostering Programme – improving the well-being of children in care through a group intervention for foster carers: study protocol for a randomised controlled trial. *Trials*, 22, 841. doi:10.1186/s13063-021-05739-y.

Perry, B. & Hambrick, E. (2008). The neurosequential model of therapeutics. *Reclaiming Children and Youth*, 17 (3), 38–43.

Redfern, S., Pursch, B., Katangwe-Chigama, T., Sopp, R., Irvine, K., Sprecher, E., Schwaiger, T., & Midgley, N. (2023). The Reflective Fostering Programme — adapting a group parenting programme for online delivery in response to the COVID-19 pandemic in the United Kingdom. *Psychology and Psychotherapy: Theory, Research and Practice*, 97 (S1), 16–30. doi:10.1111/papt.12497.

Redfern, S., Wood, S., Lassri, D., Cirasola, A., West, G., Austerberry, C., Luyten, P., Fonagy, P., & Midgley, N. (2018). The Reflective Fostering Programme (RFP): background and development of the approach. *Adoption and Fostering*, 42 (3), 234–248.

UK Government. (2023). Main findings: Children's social care in England 2023. www.gov.uk/government/statistics/childrens-social-care-data-in-england-2023/main-findings-childrens-social-care-in-england-2023.

Chapter 14

Concluding remarks

Clinical adaptations of the mentalization-based treatment model for children in the context of developmental trauma

Emma Morris, Nick Midgley and Nicole Muller

By its very nature, the question of how our own experiences may be impacted by the presence (or absence) of other minds is at the heart of developmental or attachment trauma. For children, any frightening and potentially over-whelming experience requires another mind to help make sense of what has happened; and when this is not available, it is likely that the experience cannot be fully processed. The sense of being alone, without the presence of another mind to help make sense of it, is at the heart of all traumatic experiences.

It is not surprising, therefore, that practitioners often ask about the role that mentalization-based treatment (MBT) can play in the treatment of those who have experienced trauma. In adult psychotherapy, this has led to the development of MBT-Trauma Focused (MBT-TF; Bateman et al., 2023, 277–297; Smits et al., 2024), a specific, manualized version of MBT for adults with complex PTSD, which uses a combination of psychoeducation and group intervention. When thinking about therapy with school-age children, the need to think about how a mentalization-based approach can be adapted in the context of trauma is equally important. However in this book our aim was not to present a single model of "trauma-focused MBT-C", but rather to bring together a range of ways in which practitioners have drawn on menta-lization-based approaches to inform their way of working with children, as well as their carers and the wider network around the child. This book does not offer a single recipe for this work, but rather provides a range of approaches, supported by detailed, clinical material.

In editing this book, however, it became apparent to us that there are certain over-arching principles that inform the wide range of interventions described. It was also apparent that this approach is not completely different from "core" MBT work but is better seen as an elaboration or a refinement of that model. Many of the basic principles of MBT can be applied in cases of developmental trauma. As the stories of treatment described throughout this book illustrate, the transdiagnostic, relational nature of the approach often makes it a good "fit" in these cases. Yet over the course of the chapters, we believe that certain themes emerge as key to working with developmental trauma in school-age children. These include: (a) prioritizing safety and

DOI: 10.4324/9781032713441-19

working with the child's network, (b) multi-dimensional assessment, (c) a focus on the building blocks of mentalizing and establishing epistemic trust, (d) working with avoidance and dissociative strategies, (e) focusing on the trauma-narrative in the context of the child's life story, and (f) recognizing the impact of the work on the therapist. Adapting MBT to work with children who have experienced developmental trauma often involves "turning up the volume" on these components of the model.

Prioritizing safety and working with the child's network

For children who have experienced developmental trauma, the most potent context for healing is within the caregiving relationship. When the home environment is secure enough, developmental trauma can be processed. What is needed to make this possible involves a careful assessment of the relationship between children and their carers. Vliegen and Malberg (Chapter 2) describe how to start the treatment by meeting the parents where they are and listening for their "ghosts and angels in the nursery". When parents are traumatized themselves, it can be valuable to do an assessment that includes asking about their own adverse childhood experiences and conducting a semi-structured interview such as the Parent Development Interview (PDI), as described in Chapter 3. To understand the dynamics in the carer-child relationship, some sort of live observation of play or a play-like activity such as the Squiggle game can help to identify possible frightening, dissociative, intrusive or hostile behaviour on the part of the carers. Jennifer, the mother described in Chapter 3, had been emotionally, physically, and sexually abused in her youth, and had been in a violent relationship with the father of her children. However, when she came to the assessment with her son, they were in a shelter, a safe place for them. The assessment further suggested that she was able to provide a safe enough haven for her child, both physically and psychologically, which could enable the therapeutic work to go ahead. However, when distressing mental states remain consistently not adequately mirrored, as may be the case where carers have on-going issues which may interfere with their ability to provide a safe haven for the child, a family-based approach may be indicated. In Chapter 9, Salo provides an example of how such an intervention may take place.

Sometimes a child and their carers have to be separated to restore safety for the child. In cases of ongoing abuse with highly distorted or intrusive mirroring, or neglect, where the child may also be physically at risk, there is a lack of safety. Children in these situations, with carers who are not able to make the necessary changes, will usually not engage with mentalization-based treatment and often present with highly controlling or avoidant behaviours. In these cases, the goal is to create a safe base for the child via fostering, adoptive or institutional care, and to use this relational context to mitigate the impact of relational trauma on the child to restore mentalizing capacity.

Therapy cannot proceed in cases where the developmental trauma is ongoing, and there is no "safe haven" for the child to return to. For children who are receiving ongoing care that is not safe, and for whom epistemic mistrust is protective, work in this area will be at best unsuccessful and at worst harmful, as reducing mistrust runs the risk of stripping the child of a strategy that is protecting their core self.

When a child has experienced developmental trauma, helping the network of adults around them to understand the mind and inner states behind the behaviour is of crucial importance. It is a theme that arises throughout every chapter of this book. The therapist works to help the network to mentalize the impact of the trauma on the child's development and current functioning. In doing so the therapist gives meaning to the child's behaviour; as survival behaviour that is being used out of context. With this understanding carers and others in the child's network (for example schoolteachers), if they are stuck, can be helped to move out of non-mentalizing modes and into a more compassionate, curious response. Yurko, The Ukrainian boy in the Netherlands described by Dobrova-Krol and Muller (Chapter 7) had a lot of difficulties at school. The therapist used psychoeducation and introduced the idea of "invisible luggage" to help his network understand the ongoing impact of trauma, both on his sense of safety and on his ability to understand himself and others. This helped them give a different meaning to his aggressive behaviour and resistance to engaging in school life and therefore to respond in a more attuned way. The benefits of promoting mentalization in the network around the child, and of providing psychoeducation about the impact of trauma on children and carers, is also illustrated by Redfern and Midgley's description of the Reflective Fostering Programme in the UK (Chapter 13).

In Morris's interview with Ms C. (Chapter 11), an adoptive mother describes the impact of caring for a severely traumatized child on herself and the secondary trauma she experienced as a result of hearing the details of her daughter's abuse. She describes feeling powerless, sad and alone with these feelings, and explains how having a therapist working with her alongside the sessions with her daughter, empathizing and helping her to mentalize and process her experiences, helped her to mentalize herself and her daughter better. This interview is a powerful testament to the impact that an adoptive parent can have on their child, even one who has suffered early abuse and maltreatment; as well as to the importance of working with both the child and their carer in trying to overcome the impact of developmental trauma.

Multi-dimensional assessment

Some children have experienced multiple traumas and each can have a compounding effect. In therapy, each type of trauma a child has experienced will need careful examination in order to understand how it relates to the child's development and what should be prioritized in terms of treatment. For example, if a child who has lived through war is paralysed by flashbacks and nightmares relating to what they saw, a therapist may choose to initially focus on supporting the child to manage the impact of these experiences, and only later attend to the broader impact of developmental trauma.

Another complexity with regard to assessment is often around diagnosis. In particular, the significant overlap between symptoms of autistic spectrum disorder (ASD), attention deficit hyperactivity disorder (ADHD), and developmental trauma can cause confusion. Sometimes symptoms of developmental trauma are labelled as ASD or ADHD and vice versa. It is important to keep an open mind with regard to diagnosis and the possibility that some children who have experienced developmental trauma are also neurodiverse, and that some neurodivergent children have also experienced developmental trauma.

The case of Michael (Chapter 2), a foster child who had experienced severe trauma, is a good example of how developmental trauma can have a broad ranging impact across emotional and behavioural functioning. More specifically, the chapter describes how developmental trauma has impacted on Michael's development of basic executive functioning and capacities, including stress regulation, attention, focus and learning. The chapter goes on to describe the associated problems he has in attuning and responding to foster carers and peers. These are difficulties which could easily be mistaken for symptoms of ADHD or ASD, and a differential diagnosis is sometimes needed, given that similar symptoms can sometimes have different causes.

The importance of including carers in the process of assessment with developmental trauma has already been described. Where carers have experienced trauma themselves, it is important to also assess the impact and severity of this on their parenting capacities. When possible, parents are supported to understand the impact of their trauma on their current parental and mentalizing skills, and, where appropriate, to be helped with this.

It has already been highlighted that social and cultural resources, social integration, cohesiveness and community support can have a significant impact on a parent's capacity to provide a safe relational and developmental context for their child. Despite this, many therapists tend to focus on the immediate interaction between parent and child, exploring narratives around intergenerational trauma and drawing on dyadic conceptual frameworks around attachment when making assessments. This is not necessarily inappropriate, but it is partial. The impact of systemic factors such as poverty, racism, marginalization and community support are often overlooked in assessment and their impact is not sufficiently thought about within treatment planning. A parent's mentalizing capacity may benefit far more from increased social support and improved housing conditions than by hours in the therapy room.

This was the case with Isidora's mother (Chapter 4), an immigrant mother in Chile without social network in a country where she felt lonely and isolated. Due to her own traumatic experiences, including being torn between two children because she had to leave her oldest child behind in her mother-land due to poverty, she experienced a constant heightened arousal level and a high level of epistemic mistrust. The therapist helped her to become aware of her own feelings, the impact of her life circumstances and her current, practical needs in addition to improving her understanding of her child, to become a safe and loving mother again.

A focus on the building blocks and epistemic trust

Another theme that emerges across the chapters in this book is the impor-tance of adopting a pace and focus that places the therapeutic relationship at the centre and prioritizes building trust as a therapeutic aim. Once there is confidence that a child is in a safe caregiving situation, the priority and starting point is almost always the establishment of epistemic trust with traumatized children and their families. Most children have lost trust in social knowledge and with this rigidity in their capacity to learn can emerge. The child finds it difficult to change because they cannot accept new information as trustworthy or relevant to other social contexts. Through consistent, empathic interactions, and a focus on both implicit and explicit mentalizing, children learn that others can offer helpful, reliable support, and they hope-fully begin to feel safe in exploring their own emotions and mental states. This foundational trust is critical to the child's recovery and ongoing devel-opment, as it opens them to the on-going possibility of social learning, beyond what they may learn directly from therapy.

Because of the impact of trauma on the development of epistemic trust and mentalizing capacity, and because the child often carries so many unprocessed bodily memories, particular attention is usually paid to the body in therapy with those who have experienced developmental trauma. The aim is to help the child connect with their body and bodily sensations, and promote the establishment of joint attention. Even if the child presents as seemingly very competent and engages well with the therapist, there is the possibility that this compliance may reflect a kind of pretend mode, another survival strategy. If so, the therapist should begin by focusing on the building blocks of menta-lizing, with attention control and emotion regulation via playful, physical and sensory activities. We see this process through many of the chapters in the book, including the case of Pamir (Chapter 6). Pamir found it difficult to end the therapy and expressed this by naming the pain he was feeling in different parts of his body. The therapist understood this as his way of expressing the emotional pain he felt in ending the therapy and having to say goodbye. She continued to attend to the bodily pain, enquiring about its intensity, taking Pamir's words seriously and validating his way of expressing his mental states. A similar principle holds when working with traumatized carers, where the therapist tries to build epistemic trust via empathic validation and getting alongside the carer. This was the case with Mr Brown (Chapter 10). Thinking about ways to reach out to these parents is helpful to build epistemic trust: this could involve meeting online, paying a home-visit or writing a letter after the assessment to explain how the therapist has mentalized about the family and their child. When seen as a serious attempt to reach out and connect with the family, this can sometimes open the door to collaboration.

Avoidance and dissociative strategies

The prevalence of avoidance and dissociative strategies in those who have experienced developmental trauma makes it necessary to actively look at what is not talked about or played out in therapy. These different parts of the child's experiences are of course connected but children learn to cope by becoming unaware of the connections. Because of this, children (and carers) may have a flashback to a memory, a feeling, a behaviour or a physical pain in therapy without understanding why or what triggered it. This may be very evident, or more subtle, for example with the child becoming distracted, disruptive or seemingly bored. These things are easy for the therapist and the network around the child to miss or misunderstand. The therapist may notice dissociation or avoidance early on in therapy, but may choose not to address it directly till later on, prioritizing emotion regulation and the establishment of epistemic trust in the first instance. Once a trusting relationship is established, they might engage with these processes more actively by identifying triggers and gently pursuing avoided affects, memories and thoughts. However, the therapist should quickly revert back to the focus on building epistemic trust when there is a risk that the child will move too far outside their zone of tolerance. We see this with Taro (Chapter 5) who had been neglected and both physically and sexually abused. When he shows a sexual interaction between two monster figures in his play, the therapist pleaded, "Oh, please help, it's scary!" But Taro didn't seem to hear her and continued to violently stab the zombie with a blank dissociative face. The therapist called Taro's name again. Startled, he replied "Oh, what? ... Did something happen?" Then he whispered, "You should pretend you didn't see anything." Interactions such as this one, which may occur in the context of play, can offer a an opportunity to explore the impact of trauma, not only for "the zombie in the play" but for anyone, including the therapist. Connecting with the reality of things can be challenging but is necessary if trauma is to be processed, for example by asking a child if they have ever experienced the feelings or events that are the focus of the play.

Focusing on the trauma narrative

As with all trauma-based work, development of a narrative about the trauma is central to helping both carers and children process and integrate their experiences. In this way the trauma memories can be stored differently, and the therapy can address mis-attributions, for example around blame and responsibility. With developmental trauma, because it often involves multiple traumatic experiences over a period of time, it can be important not only to identify and process key events, but also to put this in context for the child by developing a broader, coherent narrative about the traumatic relationship(s). For example a child like Taro in Chapter 5, who was neglected by his birth mother and exposed to domestic violence may need help to understand specific incidents, but may also need help to develop a story that helps them understand why their birth mother did not care for them or protect them. Not only does this help them to process and integrate traumatic feelings and experiences, it supports them in the development of a coherent autobiographical narrative and self-construct. In mentalization-based treatment this is often done initially in displacement via play, but ideally it becomes possible to put the pieces of the puzzle together more explicitly in an account that relates directly to the child's experience.

The repetitive, coercive and serious nature of Yurko's hide-and-seek game (Chapter 7) suggested a deeper traumatic meaning. He would agitatedly run away or hide, often reversing roles and repeating these actions. Given Yurko's experiences of war, it seemed that he was reenacting traumatic events. In mentalization-based treatment with traumatized children we are looking for ways to connect the play to their real experiences. Sometimes this can happen in the play itself by considering together a different ending, in which a child can feel safe or feel the power to change whatever happened to him. Sometimes it can be done in a more explicit way, as it was with Isidora (Chapter 4), who takes a baby and says that "the baby feels like vomiting", and the therapist asks her if she felt like the baby when her father forced her to eat broccoli.

Narrative work with parents can involve identifying traumatic experiences from their past which are being triggered or re-enacted in the present carer–child interaction. This includes consideration of how emotions linked with early trauma experiences can be triggered in their interaction with the child, resulting in a breakdown in mentalization. This process is described in the case of Sharon (Chapter 10) who, during a session with her mother, spoke about her being very angry and abusive. Sharon's mother froze in the moment. The therapist talked about what had happened in the next session. The mother said that the sudden openness of Sharon had triggered a painful memory of her youth when she trusted a school counsellor and told her about the sexual abuse by her brother. This resulted in an intervention where mother was taken to a crisis centre without any explanation. After Sharon's mother had shared her feelings and thoughts with the therapist she could mentalize the effect of her state of mind and behaviour on her daughter, becoming quiet, absorbed in her own feelings of panic and traumatic memories and absent in the relation with Sharon. Looking for trauma-informed patterns can help carers to change in the here and now.

Impact on the therapist

Therapists can find it disorientating to be with children who have experienced developmental trauma. For these children, movement, reflexive reaction without thinking has often taken precedence in the face of danger or unmet needs. Physical action precedes cognitive and emotional responses and trauma-related stimuli trigger sensorimotor systems that are focused on threat and danger responses that match experiences in the past. The child senses body signals and acts on them immediately, often in a teleological or psychic equivalent mode, or protects themselves by becoming disconnected. Because of this, therapists can often find themselves feeling disconnected, anxious, distressed, disgusted, frustrated, angry or confused in ways that are difficult to understand and which may lead them to a non-mentalizing response. A common response to stories about trauma is to turn your head away, close your eyes and ears, not wanting to look at it, hear about it or feel about it. However, in therapy we have to do the reverse. Finding a balance between being open, being present, being able to mentalize, being creative and at the same time not being too overwhelmed or hurt by the processes in the therapeutic relationship with traumatized children or carers is a challenge. Being authentic, a core element of the MBT stance, means the therapist stays open to the mental states of the other and to their own mental states. However, it can be challenging to stay present in the moment, let yourself be touched and to express this as much as you can in a mentalized way. A team in which the professional can feel safe to share all the strong feelings, thoughts and actions, "to think together", is necessary to achieve this balance. An external supervisor can also be helpful in dealing with the way that the impact of trauma gets played out across the wider professional network and professionals. This is especially important when the case material is personally relevant, as it was for colleague Dobrova-Krol (Chapter 7), a Ukrainian Dutch psychotherapist working with Ukrainian refugee families, feeling strongly involved in the sorrow of the families she worked with, because her motherland was also at war.

Domon-Archambault and Terradas (Chapter 12) describe a child welfare department becoming trained in a mentalization-based approach, learning to talk and think together within the same framework and therefore coming to provide a safe place for professionals and children to mentalize together. Having others to mentalize with at your work setting, in addition to engaging with good self-care and management of bodily stress outside of work, is considered a requirement in MBT, and a necessity when working with trauma.

MBT across culture

The children and families described in this book are from a range of cultural contexts, and each chapter brings with it a "taste" of that culture. For example, there are differences in the way emotions are located (for example internally versus externally) and spoken about. Olhaberry, from Chile (Chapter 4), describes how she helps Isidora to recognize the feelings inside her: "I comment, 'It seems like you were happy that we could play again'." Taro and his therapist, from Japan (Chapter 5), use more non-specific emotional expressions such as "there's some tense-feeling", which articulates the presence of an emotion without attributing it to a specific individual. This allows the therapist and child to share the same emotional space, even though each person may have a different kind of engagement with that feeling. Many factors, including a person's socio-economic background, religion, ability, age, sexuality, gender and family culture, influence the way they feel, express and give meaning to emotions (Mesquita, 2022).

While the parenting practices, interpretation of behaviour and affective responses of the families and therapists described in this book are heavily influenced by different social and cultural constructs, values and norms, the contributing authors are working towards a shared aim: To strengthen mentalizing in families, with the belief that this will lead to greater capacity for emotion regulation, for building strong and supportive relationships, for promoting a sense of self and the capacity to engage in social learning. The emphasis on curiosity, uncertainty and non-judgement adopted by MBT practitioners, which sits well with a position of cultural humility, in addition to the focus on social learning allows for a level of cultural flexibility. In this sense it could be argued that MBT is not only a trans-diagnostic model, but also trans-cultural one. However, much more work is needed to truly understand the role of mentalizing across cultures, as well as to understand to what degree mentalization-based treatments need to be adapted to suit the needs of children and families in different settings.

References

Bateman, A., Fonagy, P., Campbell, C., Luyten, P., & Debbané, M. (2023). *Cambridge guide to mentalization-based treatment (MBT)*. Cambridge Guides to the Psychological Therapies. Cambridge University Press.

Mesquita, B. (2022). *Between us: How cultures create emotions*. Norton and Co.

Smits, M. L., de Vos, J., Rüfenacht, E., Nijssens, L., Shaverin, L., Nolte, T., Luyten, P., Fonagy, P., & Bateman, A. (2024). Breaking the cycle with trauma-focused mentalization-based treatment: theory and practice of a trauma-focused group intervention. *Frontiers of Psychology*, 13 (15), 1426092. doi:10.3389/fpsyg.2024.1426092.

Glossary of mentalizing terms

This glossary was developed with the support of CoPilot AI software.

Affect regulation   See "Emotion regulation".

Agency   In mentalization theory, agency refers to the sense of being the originator of one's own actions and having control over one's thoughts, feelings, and behaviours. It involves recognizing oneself as an active participant in shaping one's experiences and interactions with the world.

Alien self   In MBT, the concept of the "alien self" refers to parts of the self that feel foreign or not truly integrated into one's identity. This often occurs when early attachment relationships fail to adequately mirror and validate a child's emotional experiences. As a result, these unacknowledged or poorly understood parts of the self can feel alien or disconnected.

Attention control   Attention control refers to an individual's ability to choose what they pay attention to and what they ignore, both in terms of physical experience and sensations, and mental states (emotions, thoughts etc.). This skill is crucial for focusing on relevant tasks while filtering out distractions. In MBT it is considered one of the "building blocks" (see below) of the capacity to mentalize.

Building blocks of mentalization   The capacity to mentalize, or understand and interpret one's own and others' mental states, is built on several key components – these are referred to as the "building

DOI: 10.4324/9781032713441-20

blocks" of mentalizing. These building blocks work together to help individuals navigate social interactions and understand the mental states that drive behaviour. They include: (1) attention control (the ability to focus and sustain attention on relevant stimuli while ignoring distractions); (2) emotion regulation (the capacity to manage and respond to one's emotional experiences); (3) explicit mentalization (the ability to consciously reflect on and understand one's own and others' thoughts, feelings, and intentions).

Congruent mirroring

In mentalization theory, congruent mirroring refers to the process where a caregiver accurately reflects the emotional state of the infant in a way that matches the infant's internal experience. This mirroring helps the child understand and regulate their own emotions by seeing them accurately reflected and acknowledged by the caregiver.

Contingent mirroring

Contingent mirroring in mentalization theory refers to the process where a caregiver responds to an infant's emotional expressions in a way that is both accurate and timely. This means the caregiver's response is directly related to the infant's current emotional state, helping the infant to recognize and understand their own emotion.

Dimensions of mentalizing

Mentalizing involves several key components that help individuals understand and interpret their own and others' mental states. These components work together to enable a comprehensive understanding of mental states, which is crucial for effective social interactions and emotional regulation. The four components are considered to be: (1) automatic vs. controlled (mentalizing can occur automatically, without conscious effort, or in a controlled, deliberate manner); (2) self vs. other (this dimension involves understanding one's own mental states as well as those of others); (3) inner vs. outer (mentalizing includes interpreting internal mental states (thoughts, feelings) and external behaviours); and (4) cognitive vs. affective (this involves both cognitive processes (thinking about thoughts) and affective processes (understanding emotions)).

Embodied mentalizing

Embodied mentalizing refers to the process of understanding and interpreting one's own and others' mental states through non-verbal, physical actions and bodily expressions. This concept emphasizes that mentalizing can occur not just through verbal communication but also through gestures, facial expressions, and other forms of body language.

Emotion regulation

In mentalization theory, emotion regulation refers to the ability to manage and respond to one's emotional experiences in a healthy and adaptive way. This involves recognizing, understanding, and modulating emotions to maintain emotional stability and well-being. Effective emotion regulation is considered one of the "building blocks" of the capacity to mentalize, and allows individuals to reflect on their emotions without becoming overwhelmed by them. This capacity helps in understanding both one's own and others' mental states, which is essential for healthy interpersonal relationships and overall mental health.

Empathic validation

Empathic validation in MBT involves the therapist acknowledging and reflecting the client's emotional state in a way that shows understanding and acceptance. This process helps to stabilize the client's sense of self and reduce anxiety by demonstrating that the therapist sees things from the client's perspective.

Epistemic hypervigilance

Epistemic hypervigilance refers to an excessive and heightened state of alertness towards the trustworthiness of information and the intentions of others. This state often results from past relational traumas or inconsistent caregiving, leading individuals to be overly cautious and sceptical about the information they receive. In a state of epistemic hypervigilance, the receiver of communication assumes that the intentions of the person communicating are different from those openly expressed. Most characteristic is the assumption of bad intentions underlying other people's actions.

Epistemic mistrust

Epistemic mistrust refers to a lack of trust in the knowledge and information communicated by others. This mistrust can make it difficult for individuals to accept and integrate new information, which is crucial for social learning and therapeutic progress. Epistemic mistrust often arises from negative past experiences, such as trauma or inconsistent caregiving, leading individuals to be wary of others' intentions and the validity of the information they provide. In MBT, addressing epistemic mistrust involves creating a safe and validating therapeutic environment to help rebuild trust in interpersonal communication.

Epistemic trust

Epistemic trust refers to the capacity to trust the knowledge and information communicated by others as relevant, significant, and applicable to oneself. This trust is crucial for effective social learning and therapeutic progress.

Explicit mentalizing

Explicit mentalizing refers to the conscious, reflective process of understanding and interpreting one's own and others' mental states. Unlike implicit mentalizing, which is automatic and non-conscious, explicit mentalizing involves deliberate thought and awareness.

Marked mirroring

Marked mirroring in mentalization theory refers to the process where a caregiver reflects an infant's emotional state in a way that is both accurate and clearly distinguished from the caregiver's own emotions. This involves the caregiver responding to the infant's emotions with exaggerated, yet appropriate, facial expressions and tones that signal to the infant that the caregiver understands their feeling.

Mentalizing	Mentalizing is the ability to understand and interpret one's own and others' mental states, such as thoughts, feelings, intentions, and desires. This skill helps individuals make sense of their own behaviour and the behaviour of others, facilitating effective social interactions and emotional regulation.
Mentalized affectivity	Mentalized affectivity refers to the ability to understand and manage one's emotions by reflecting on them and their underlying causes.
Mentalizing profile	A mentalizing profile refers to an individual or family's unique pattern of strengths and weaknesses in their ability to mentalize, or understand and interpret their own and others' mental states. This profile can help therapists tailor interventions to better support the individual or family's specific needs in therapy.
Mentalizing stance	The mentalizing stance is an attitude in which an individual actively seeks to understand and reflect on the mental states – such as thoughts, feelings, intentions, beliefs, and desires – of themselves and others. It involves recognizing that behaviour is not random but is shaped by these internal mental states. This stance is central to the process of mentalizing, which is the ability to make sense of human behaviour by imagining the inner worlds of oneself and others. Curiosity, perspective-taking and being nonjudgmental are core aspects of the mentalizing stance.
Mirroring	Mirroring in mentalization refers to the process where a caregiver reflects an infant's emotional state back to them through facial expressions, tone of voice, and body language. This helps the infant recognize and understand their own emotions, which is crucial for developing the capacity to mentalize. These processes help the infant develop a sense of their own mental states and lay the foundation for understanding others' mental states as well.

There are different types of mirroring: (1) congruent mirroring (accurately reflecting the infant's emotional state); (2) contingent mirroring (responding to the infant's emotions in a timely and appropriate manner); and (3) marked mirroring (reflecting the infant's emotions in a way that is clearly distinguished from the caregiver's own emotions, often using exaggerated expressions).

Not-knowing stance
This aspect of the therapeutic stance revolves around a willingness to know more about the client's mind, combined with a certain humility due to the awareness of not being able to know exactly what is going on in the other person (the opacity of minds).

Ostensive cues
Signals by which a person communicates to another that what they want to convey is relevant. These include eye contact, raised eyebrows, special voice use or personalised content, such as explicitly mentioning the child's name. This makes the other feel recognised as a person in their own right which creates openness and builds epistemic confidence. These ostensive cues can vary in different cultures.

Parental reflective functioning
Parental reflective functioning (PRF) refers to a caregiver's ability to understand and reflect upon their own and their child's internal mental states, such as thoughts, feelings, and intentions. This capacity is crucial for fostering a child's emotional development, secure attachment, and ability to mentalize, which means understanding behaviour in terms of underlying mental states, By effectively engaging in PRF, caregivers help children develop better emotion regulation, a sense of personal agency, and healthier social relationships.

Pre-mentalizing modes
Pre-mentalizing modes are ways of thinking and interacting that occur when the capacity to mentalize is disrupted or underdeveloped. These modes are typically seen in early childhood but can reappear in problematic ways in later life, especially

when under stress. Understanding these modes helps in identifying when someone is struggling with mentalizing and provides a framework for therapeutic interventions. The three main pre-mentalizing modes are: (1) teleological mode (this mode focuses on physical actions and outcomes rather than mental states – people in this mode believe that only observable actions and their results are real and meaningful); psychic equivalence mode (in this mode, internal and external realities are seen as identical – Individuals believe that their thoughts and feelings are directly reflective of reality, leading to difficulties in distinguishing between subjective experiences and objective facts); and (3) pretend mode (here, mental states are decoupled from reality. Individuals might engage in fantasy or intellectualization, where their thoughts and feelings are disconnected from real-life situations).

Pretend mode   See "Pre-mentalizing modes".

Psychic equivalence mode   See "Pre-mentalizing modes".

Reflective functioning   Reflective functioning refers to the ability to understand and interpret one's own and others' mental states, such as thoughts, feelings, and intentions. This capacity is crucial for effective social interactions and emotional regulation. The term is sometimes used interchangeably with "mentalizing", or can be considered as an operationalisation of mentalizing ability, i.e. how the capacity to mentalize is measured.

Self   In mentalization theory, the self is understood as a dynamic and evolving construct that emerges from the ability to mentalize, or understand and interpret one's own and others' mental states. The development of a stable and coherent self is closely linked to secure attachment relationships and the ability to mentalize effectively. When individuals can accurately understand and reflect on their own and others' mental

	states, they develop a stronger sense of identity and personal agency.
Social learning	In mentalization theory, social learning refers to the process by which individuals learn about their own and others' mental states through social interactions. This involves observing and interpreting the behaviours, emotions, and intentions of others, which helps in understanding and predicting social behaviour. Mentalization theory emphasizes the importance of understanding the mental states that underlie observable actions, which is crucial for effective social functioning and empathy.
Teleological mode	See "Pre-mentalizing mode".
Under-developed mentalizing	Under developed mentalizing refers to a limited ability to understand and interpret one's own and others' mental states, such as thoughts, feelings, and intentions. Individuals with under-developed mentalizing may struggle to direct and focus their attention. They also struggle with recognizing emotions, have difficulty identifying and labelling their own and others' emotions, understanding behaviour and regulating emotions.
We-mode	In MBT, "we mode" refers to a therapeutic stance where both the therapist and the client collaboratively focus on understanding the client's mental states and their interactions with others. The mere presence of others creates the possibility for developing shared perspectives. Co-representing the viewpoints of others and generating a "psychological collective" by joining forces, can lead to an emerging sense of "we-ness", of shared perspectives and shared minds, which is at the heart of relational mentalizing.

Index

For Product Safety Concerns and Information please contact our EU
representative GPSR@taylorandfrancis.com
Taylor & Francis Verlag GmbH, Kaufingerstraße 24, 80331 München, Germany